Back on Track

Dedication

This book is dedicated to my parents, Robyn and Gary, my partner Steve and a small army of friends for their amazing support. Thank you for the positivity and help you all brought to a lengthy but successful recovery process.

Credits

Zoe Catchpole

Tania Cotton

Steve Hobson

Kate McCombe

Dave Scott

Neil MacClean-Martin

Tremay Dobson

Oliver Weber

Chris Fidler

Paul Newsome

Rachel Morris

Claire Cameron

Karin Cannons

David Lane

Steve Trew

Kelvin Wright

Kerrie O'Connor

Chris Taylor

Ryan Gregson

Genevieve LaCaze

Jimmy May

Susan Lunn

Bethan Jones

Zoe Wafelbakker

Marina Lim

Caroline Hermon

Nancy Doherty

Aidan Prior

Deborah Pearson

Frank O'Connor

FIONA FORD

INTERNATIONAL TRIATHLETE

BACK ON TRACK

HOW I RECOVERED FROM A LIFE-CHANGING
ACCIDENT AND GOT BACK ON THE PODIUM

Meyer & Meyer Sport

British Library Cataloguing in Publication Data
A catalogue record for this book is available from the British Library

**Back on Track – How I recovered from a life-changing
accident and got back on the podium**
Maidenhead: Meyer & Meyer Sport (UK) Ltd., 2015
ISBN: 978-1-78255-074-7

© 2015 by Meyer & Meyer Sport (UK) Ltd.
Aachen, Auckland, Beirut, Cairo, Cape Town, Dubai, Hägendorf, Hong Kong,
Indianapolis, Manila, New Delhi, Singapore, Sydney, Tehran, Vienna
Member of the World Sport Publishers' Association (WSPA)
Manufacturing: Print Consult GmbH, Munich, Germany
ISBN: 978-1-78255-074-7
E-Mail: info@m-m-sports.com
www.m-m-sports.com

TABLE OF CONTENTS

PREFACE

Endurance, n

Definition: The fact of enduring (pain, hardship, annoyance); the habit or the power of enduring; often absol. as denoting a quality, longsuffering, patience.

Oxford English Dictionary

The year of the London 2012 Olympics I had enjoyed over a decade in the sport of triathlon, transitioning from marathon runner into multisport. While teaching in Poplar, East London, I ran the London marathon a number of times earning a championship start time and encouraging my pupils to take up (any) sport. One of my students, Perri Shakes-Drayton, competed at the London 2012 Olympics. To watch her race a decade on from challenging me to races up and down the school playground was an absolute pleasure. On marathon day in 2003, as a 12 year old, Perri ran the length of Poplar High Street with me as the route passed by the school gates. I appreciated her positive attitude as I managed and taught a challenging class the year I decided to run my last London marathon.

Embracing triathlon in 2002, I raced for Great Britain in age group teams at ITU World Championships for 4 years, culminating with winning 'double', the Aquathlon and Triathlon in the same week. I finished third and fifth overall respectively in the women's age group events, a few minutes behind Chrissie Wellington in the ITU Triathlon when all the age group results were amalgamated together.

With the support of a bike sponsor, Planet-X, and coached by Spencer Smith, I was encouraged to turn to long course triathlon racing. My first Ironman® event in 2007 was ® France. I finished in the top 10 overall, setting a new age group course record and qualifying for the World Championships in Kona, Hawaii. I finished top 10 in my age group after injuring myself in the early stages of the race taking evasive action to avoid a crash on the road outside the transition between swim and bike. I still managed to run a sub 3:30 marathon off the bike, always relishing the ability to harness discomfort in the familiar rhythm of endurance running.

Over the next four years I trained consistently and raced in the pro ranks producing Ironman® top 10 finishes while also working full time.

In 2010 I made the leap of faith to set up a full-time coaching business, leaving the security of my role as an educational consultant. I naively expected that doing what I loved full time would provide me with a more optimal training focus. However, if anything, more time was required in the first 2-3 years setting up a business from scratch. Time was preciously unavailable for me to invest in logging training hours. A quality over quantity approach prevailed.

In 2009 and 2010 I produced two sub 10 hour Ironman® finishes. I was averaging 13 hours training per week due to putting in 60 hours work! My race calendar in the season featured just a handful of events to peak for as a result. In 2011 I experimented with racing back-to-back Ironman® events just 4 weeks apart. As a coach I sought to gain insight into the leanest possible timescale of a standard recovery process. I finished fourth at Challenge Vichy and tenth at Challenge Henley, earning prize money at each event I raced.

In 2012 I was keen to make a podium at an Ironman® event and had made tough decisions to improve key aspects in my life that were having a significantly negative impact on my well-being. As a result of making one difficult change, my training had responded better than ever to an altitude training block in the alps with my coached athletes. I had mapped out a season ahead of me and was eager to make the next leap in performance to a step on the podium. My business was becoming nicely established and I hoped to bring some balance into the work–training–life equation in 2012 to race up another level.

And then on an ordinary weekend training ride, on an ordinary British summer day, against the backdrop of the country's finest year of cycling, a car knocked me off my bike.

I snapped my right collarbone, shattered my pelvis, broke my sacrum and fractured some vertebrae. I grazed off approximately half a metre of skin. My helmet shattered down the middle leaving a long, large lump on the side of my head, cutting off my hair in the same place. The impact was so intense that I wore the rectangular imprint of my iPhone on the skin and flesh on the side of my back like branding for six months.

I was told I would never be able to run again, never be able to do a marathon. I feared I would never be able to walk.

In the two to three seconds it took for my body to smash into the tarmac at 35 kph everything changed: My life altered irrevocably by a careless, thoughtless, bike-blind driver. I was left facing an endurance challenge that had ever-changing rules and a finish line that kept moving further and further away. At 1:30 pm on June 23 suffering, hardship, pain and endurance all took on a new significance.

My wonderful, extraordinary life had been turned upside down. My livelihood, home, quality of life and even the ability to look after myself independently were all under threat. I was at the bottom of an unfamiliar mountain I couldn't see a summit of – with an arduous climb ahead.

Over the past two years I have endured a lengthy process and continuous challenge. By having a new start line defined for me, unsure of the journey I would take to reach the finish, I relied on belief. Belief that I knew the direction I needed to head in and an understanding that I should aim to keep on moving toward the summit, continually climbing, however slowly.

Previously defined limits paled into insignificance compared to starting over again – teaching myself to walk, to swim, to run and to bike all over again. The journey to return to an active life again has been helped at many stages by medical professionals, physiotherapists, sports trainers, massage therapists, my coached athletes, friends, family and a supportive partner.

My greatest source of strength when the chips were down was applying principles from a previously active, athletic life to a recovery process without frustration that I could not train or wasn't racing. Having serious injuries provided an opportunity to evaluate the important things in life.

This is my personal story of my recovery from a serious bike accident and guide to making the transition from rehabilitation back to functional movement and back into training. It is intended to assist any injured active person, whether an athlete or sports enthusiast, to prepare for an event that is not clearly defined and doesn't have a finish line.

My intention by writing this book is that the reader will see that endurance, determination and consistency is rewarded not with medals and trophies or accolades but with a result that is arguably much greater.

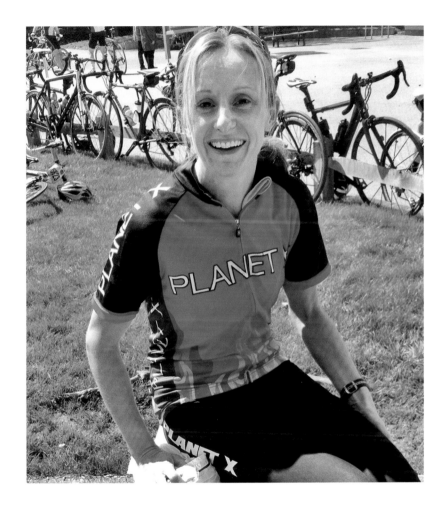

CHAPTER 1:
BICYCLE VERSUS CAR

Biggest achievement: Surviving high-speed bike crash

Top speed: 51.5 kph
Elevation gain: 797 m
Distance: 64.54 km

1:30 pm Saturday 23 June 2012

Maintaining an easy cadence and effort over the rolling hills of Surrey I regularly glanced back to check my friend Tania who was happily pedalling on my wheel. She had made light work of the Surrey hills on a trip to visit London; after all she was used to riding in her home environment of the French Alps.

We had planned a low-key training ride on the London 2012 Olympic road cycle route, taking in the Box Hill 'climb', factoring in an obligatory cake-and-coffee stop mid route. In just a few weeks the same roads would be lined with cycling-crazy fans in a year in which the UK embarked on a serious love affair with the sport thanks to a landmark Tour De France win for Bradley Wiggins.

My newly built, custom-specced race bike had proved to be a flawless ride on its third outing. I felt at one with the bike as it cruised through training miles even though I had only sat on it a handful of times. I couldn't wait to see what it could do when the summer season kicked off for my fourth year racing as a pro.

My attention turned to the increasing traffic levels around the middle of the day, and I checked on Tania again as we swooped up over the railway bridge at Oxshott. I soft-pedalled before cresting over the top of the small rise and sensed her closing down the small gap between us. My time trial bike was eager to be off and I allowed it to run a little on the slight descent, feathering the brakes lightly.

As I approached a junction I spotted a dark blue car stopped on the left waiting to turn into the road we were travelling along. I floated out into the road and stared at the driver's side window to try to make eye contact. It was a tactic I used all the time to make sure I was spotted easily by motorists. The relentless flow of oncoming traffic made me confident the driver could not and would not pull out.

But then he did. Just metres from my front wheel.

What happened in a tenth of a second all unfolded in hideous, silent slow motion. My mind quickly presented me with two options, and neither of them was great. Option A: hit the front brakes, which would mean a trip over the handlebars onto his car and then probably into the oncoming traffic. Option B: use the emergency *squeezetherearbrake* technique and hope like hell I could use my years of race-honed skills to dodge him.

My subconscious immediately chose option B. I applied the back brake and aimed the front wheel slightly towards what I hoped would present itself as a small gap as the car moved forwards. Then the rear wheel of my bike left the road, and I sensed both the bike and I were airborne. I closed my eyes when I realised the bike was out of control, and I would be taking the full impact of a high-speed crash on the right side of my body. There was nothing more I could do. It seemed a long tenth of a second.

When it came, the impact with the road was horrendous. My hip, back, right leg, left knee, right shoulder, right arm, left fingertips, right hand, head and helmet all met the tarmac, ripping the bike from under me, and I skidded along the road for some distance. One of my bike shoes remained clipped into the pedals as my right foot was yanked out of it forcefully.

I finally came to a stop in the middle of the road. When I opened my eyes I saw oncoming traffic, the wheels at eye level, pointed towards my head. Tania's shouts to the driver of the dark blue hatchback, 'stop, stop, stop!' were ringing in my ears as I lay on the road.

I heard a long groan and realised the noise had just come from me. I felt oddly disconnected from the situation as I struggled to make sense of what had just happened. My mind was overloaded with debilitating feedback coming from my crumpled body, and I recognised the signals were indicating a serious state of shock and trauma.

I knew immediately that my right collarbone had snapped, literally like a twig beneath my ear. It was, though, the least of my worries. The pain radiating in relentless waves through my body from my back and my hips was intolerable.

My head pounded inside my helmet.

I could barely control my breathing and had to try to resist the temptation to close my eyes to cope with the high levels of pain. I became aware of a sinister tingling sensation in my lower body and lack of feeling in my legs. It was then that I knew I should not move.

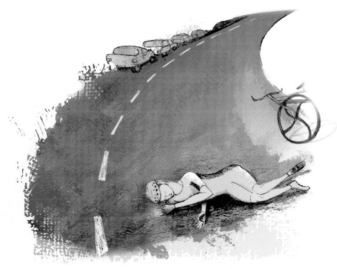

Junction of Warren Lane and Sandy Lane, Oxshott, Surrey, UK

Tania asked one of the motorists who had stopped to help to phone an ambulance. I could hear panic in her voice and wished that I could do something, but all I could do was lie in the middle of the road, feeling extremely vulnerable, and wait until help arrived. A car whizzed past dangerously close to me, impatient at the traffic slowing to a halt where I lay fallen on the road. I felt a rush of panic followed by a wave of adrenaline surge through me as I glimpsed car tyres flashing past within centimetres of my head and back.

Then my right hamstring started to go into an excruciating cramp. The flight instinct had kicked in and with it unconscious initiation of movement. No matter how hard I tried to focus on releasing the tension, the pain seemed to be an insurmountable barrier to initiating any movement in my leg at all. I begged Tania, who was now by my side, to straighten my left leg for me. She grasped my upper leg, knee and ankle and expertly helped the leg relax down on top of the right.

Then help arrived. She was called Debbie and had stopped when she had seen what had happened. Her face suddenly appeared right in front of mine, and she introduced herself then said she would help me until the ambulance arrived. Her simple act of kneeling in front of the oncoming traffic and mounting chaos around me on the road was very reassuring.

She helped me to focus on my breaths to manage the pain somewhat, and every time I attempted to close my eyes, she would lightly bring me back to the present and remind me to continue breathing in and out, with her. During this time she managed to coax from me simple facts such was who I was, where I lived, whether I knew where I was and what had happened to me.

Tania and Debbie had a brief animated conversation about how soon an ambulance would arrive, but I wasn't sure how much longer I could hold on. My eyes kept wanting to close, and I wished I could switch off the mounting pain levels. Debbie helped support my head from the hardness of the road as I lay there, and I used my left arm, slowly and painstakingly with assistance, to take some of the weight off my broken right shoulder.

From my view lying on the tarmac I could occasionally make out the legs of cyclists who were on the side of the road and had obviously stopped to assist. The kit they were wearing seemed familiar, and I tried to focus on that to distract from the pain. I was now having difficulty maintaining concentration and struggled to keep breathing in time with Debbie. Tania reassured me the ambulance was on its way.

'It is very important to gain the help of witnesses at the scene of the accident, recording their contact details in case their help or observations are needed in the future. Don't lose the small window of opportunity when other cyclists, motorists or passers-by are present.'

Tania Cotton
Health in Motion founder, movement analyst, British chartered physiotherapist

After what seemed like hours lying on the road a rapid response vehicle arrived, and the emergency care assistant assessed my situation. My relief turned to panic when he swiftly suggested that I be moved from the road because of the growing traffic jam.

The thought of being moved terrified me. My levels of pain were now off the scale. Fortunately Debbie and Tania were united and robust: no spinal board, no moving. In the end he came round to their view and agreed it was best to wait for an ambulance.

He tried to fit a breathing device to provide me with gas pain relief. It didn't work. We ran through the questions: Where are you? Who are you? What happened? Then he asked me to move my left arm from under my right shoulder because he wanted to trace where the blood on the road underneath me was coming from. Moving triggered another wave of nauseating, excruciating pain. The source of the bleeding: the skin had been scraped off my left fingertips as I skidded along the road.

Despite the warmth of a summer day I could now feel myself getting cold very quickly and noticed I had started to shake uncontrollably. It had not occurred to me to ask for something to keep me warm. Tania suggested to the emergency responder that he should find a blanket to cover me as I was going into shock.

By now my mouth was completely dry and swallowing was an effort. The athlete in me recognised that having been riding for three hours I was now in need of water or fluids. Thirst indicates that the body is already slightly dehydrated and over many years of honing fuelling strategies on long rides and runs it was efficient and automatic to drink little and often on endurance sessions. I'd gone past the point of having anything in my control and all my senses seemed on high alert. I was desperate for water.

'Individuals will react differently when it comes to managing high pain levels and uncertainty at the scene of an accident. If at all possible it is best to focus on remaining calm and breathing. Panicking, although difficult to prevent, will waste energy and make the situation more difficult for those with you to do their job, which ultimately impacts on your care. Focus on things that are important to you, friends and loved ones. Try to reassure yourself that help is on its way and that pain relief will come with that too.'

Kate McCombe, *consultant anaesthetist, Frimley Park Hospital*

Finally I saw the welcome sight of blue flashing lights on top of stripes of fluorescent colour. A large lumbering ambulance was squeezing its way along the road towards me. My eyes closed as a wave of relief passed over me. When I opened them again I saw four women medics heading in my direction armed with medical kit. Debbie slipped away after explaining she was handing over to the new arrivals. Thank you seemed such an insignificant gesture for all she had done. I would never see her again.

Six ways to help yourself in an accident, applying athlete-honed skills and principles:

1. Use your skills as a competitor to stay focused on what you can do, not on what you cannot do.

2. Draw on controlled breathing strategies used in training and racing to help you focus on staying present and controlling your pain levels.

3. Prioritise. Think about what you need and in what order.

4. Remember pain is temporary. Recall those training sessions and races where you went through the pain barrier. You are more resilient than you think.

5. Think positive. Tell yourself: 'You are alive, you survived' and avoid letting the mind think about the implications of your injuries.

6. Think family. Use thinking about your friends and family as a coping strategy to combat fear and anxiety.

I was asked to describe the pain and explained I knew I had broken my right collarbone and was worried that I could neither feel nor move my legs. They concluded I needed pain relief immediately. Finally. By the time they started to get to work I was feeling strangely disconnected from the whole scene. It was like I was watching them from above as they attempted to insert an IV drip into my arm, failing on numerous attempts because of the dehydration before considering trying to get a catheter in my foot. Either option was fine with me. I willed them to find success.

The lead medic explained I was about to be rolled onto a spinal board to move me safely into the ambulance where I could be treated. I would also have a neck brace fitted and be supported by an 'inflatable' bean bag around my legs, hips and body. At this point I sharply rejoined reality. Me, move? My broken helmet was carefully removed in preparation.

I became acutely aware of a number of people around me, and I could feel the board being slid next to me on the road. I was gripped by a moment of fear as hands were positioned along my legs, hips, back, shoulders and head. Deftly, decisively, on a count of three, I was rolled onto my back. I screamed involuntarily as I felt the indescribable pain of my bones crunching through my hips and back.

I lay there quietly looking at the sky as I felt the 'bean bag' pack out around me. A neck brace had also been fitted with difficulty, but the pain was subsiding.

A medic retrieved my phone and house keys from the pocket of my cycling jersey. I could vaguely feel heightened discomfort along my lower spine once I had been rolled. As she pulled the shattered mobile free from underneath my body she was alarmed to find it covered in a sticky dark liquid. Quickly she started to investigate before I stopped her and assured her it was not blood but, judging from the smell, one of my energy gels that must have exploded as I hit the ground. It was a much-needed moment of levity before the rear doors of the ambulance closed.

The inside of the ambulance felt surreal and calm, which was a welcome contrast from the chaos of lying injured on the road. The medics set about checking my condition and recording details. They discovered I still had one bicycle shoe on and there was some speculation as to where the other shoe was. Presumably still clipped into the pedal on my bike. I had to talk them through the complicated clasp system so they could remove it. As I couldn't feel my feet or move them, all I could do was consider how much was force required to rip a foot cleanly out of a tightly fitting bike shoe.

As we rattled along, the medics asked about what sport I did, and I explained to them what Ironman® triathlon was all about. As we continued the 20-minute journey, I tried to keep myself in the present to fend off the rising fears about what the future might hold and the implications of my injuries. All the time hanging in the air was that one question I didn't want to ask but which I knew needed to be answered. What did that sinister tingling and lack of feeling in my lower body mean?

For a fleeting moment I wondered whether I would ever ride my bike again; with Tania I had ridden many kilometres over every mountain pass in the French Alps. I recalled a few of my best world-class performances at races and the feeling of unstoppable strength and speed. I closed my eyes and absorbed the full force of my doubts as we made progress steadily towards the hospital.

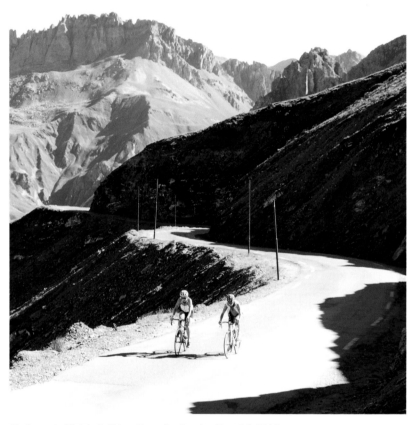

Final ascent of Col du Galibier – Route des Grandes Alpes, July 2010

Dos and don'ts

Helping a training partner at the scene of an accident:

DO:
Ensure your own personal safety before helping so you don't end up in a situation with two accident victims not just one.

Call the emergency services (999 in the UK, 112 in European Union countries). Tell the injured person the emergency services have been contacted and help is on its way

Establish if the person is breathing and conscious. If not then check the neck for the carotid pulse (this is just next to the windpipe on both sides) or the radial pulse in the wrist (use your first two fingers, not your thumb, for this).

If the person cannot breathe or is snoring gently carefully open their airway by lifting their jaw forward in a thrust to allow air into the lungs. Be careful not to move their neck. If there is something blocking the airway that can be removed easily then do so but ensure you do not push it further down.

If you can and if necessary then start basic life support with cardiopulmonary resuscitation using chest compressions.

If there are areas where a person is losing blood, apply a piece of rolled-up material firmly to the site but do not take it off to check if it's working.

If there is significant bleeding from an arm or leg, tie something, such as a belt, above the bleeding point tightly as a tourniquet.

Cover the patient up and keep them warm.

Talk to your injured friend and make them talk to you. If they are conscious they will have higher levels of adrenaline, which will help them maintain blood pressure to keep their vital organs working.

Find out the victim's full name, age, date of birth and next of kin details and ascertain if they have any medical problems or allergies. This information should be passed to the ambulance crew.

DON'T:

Show panic or stress – it's infectious and will transmit to the injured person. Take a few deep breaths before you approach and tell yourself to stay calm.

Move the patient. Only do so if they are in extreme danger. Moving someone could damage their spinal cord and risk paralysing them.

Take off their cycling helmet – for the same reasons you should not move them.

Remove any glass, metal or other objects lodged in a patient's body – it could be 'plugging a hole', and taking it out could cause bleeding.

Give the person food or drink – they may need general anaesthetic and surgery and to do so would increase the risk of a lung infection.

Source: Kate McCombe, consultant anaesthetist, and Kelvin Wright, consultant in emergency medicine and critical care, Frimley Park Hospital, Surrey.

Top four cycle safety tips:

1.   Wear or carry some form of identification containing your name, address, contact details for next of kin and important medical information. There are a number of wristbands available on the market offering a personalised way to display vital information.

2.   Plan your cycling route to avoid busy areas at peak times of day where possible. Look for quieter back roads or dedicated cycle

route roads. There are lots of apps and online data sharing sites now available to help you do this. Local cyclists will likely have established safe and scenic route options in highly populated areas.

3. Pack items into your cycling pockets safely. Sharp objects could injure your back or sides, so think about where you pack objects like mobile phones and keys. Put things that could be dangerous, CO_2 cartridges, bike pumps, tyre levers, in saddle bags or attach them to the bike frame. Pack your mobile phone in a soft case.

4. Always wear a cycling helmet

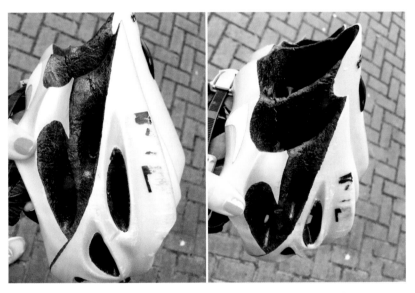

A helmet could go a long way in saving your life in a high-speed impact with the road or car

'Yesterday is past, tomorrow is another day, today is a gift. That's why it's called the present.'

CHAPTER 2:
ACCIDENT AND EMERGENCY

Biggest achievement: Successfully moved from ambulance trolley to hospital bed

Top speed: 2 kph being wheeled on hospital trolley
Elevation gain: 1.8 m in hoist for back examination
Distance: 25 km to hospital

2 pm Saturday 23 June 2012

I could feel the ambulance slowing down and carefully turning before reversing back to a halt. I had arrived at the hospital. I closed my eyes again as I felt another wave of emotion rush over me; soon I would know what damage had been inflicted by the impact.

I feared the intolerable level of pain returning although felt strangely calm about finding out the extent of my injuries. Trying to be rational, I thought at least knowing what I would be dealing with would provide me with somewhere to start. I could then put an end to the speculation and deal with the facts.

I was soon whisked out of the ambulance, cocooned in the bean bag on the trolley, and into the accident and emergency reception area. Staring at a range of different ceilings meant I hadn't a clue where I was, and there was a new team of faces making observations for treatment. Once inside a cubicle a doctor started an assessment and asked questions of the accident and what I could remember of the impact. He explained that I would need to be examined and have some tests done. First they had to get me out of the bean bag and transfer me to a different spinal board through which I could be checked over.

A small team of nurses and doctors returned, including the ambulance medics, to remove me from my bean bag haven. I cried out in pain as I was rolled carefully from side to side to remove the support. It felt very disturbing not to be able to engage with my muscles to help move my legs or lower body in any way. It was like I had been disconnected somehow through the middle. Still at least the pain medication was working, and the levels had dropped from excruciating to just about manageable if I didn't move a millimetre.

When I was returned to the cubicle, the nurses let me know they needed to cut off my cycle clothing. As with my missing bike shoe, I felt a little upset that my kit would be destroyed in the process. However I could sense a restrictive tangle of cycle clothing around my shoulders and back and accepted this wasn't a task I would be undertaking myself anytime soon.

The nurses set about slicing through my lovely white cycling gillet, team jersey, bib shorts and light base layer insulating my skin. It took some time to prise close-fitting cycling kit out from underneath me as I could move barely millimetres – and that only with great effort. The gillet provided a particular puzzle for the medical team because it had become tangled around my shoulders and upper back.

It appeared three layers of clothing had been no match for the tarmac. The back of my right shoulder felt like it had been grated once the clothing that was stuck to it was pulled away from the skin. The process of cutting through my cycle shorts was difficult and indicated how much impact the back and right side of my hip had taken when it had met the road. Even my socks and fingerless gloves had not escaped road damage. Once the nurses had fitted sensors and hooked me up to the machine monitoring vital signs, I was semi-covered in a hospital gown, and a sling was fitted to my right arm to help support the shoulder. It took what seemed an age.

I dared not move and lay still attempting to manage the discomfort from all areas of my body. I felt like a living corpse, motionless but quite stable thanks to the pain medication, IV drip and machines monitoring my breathing, temperature, heart rate and vital signs. The medical profession refers to it as 'comfortable' – it was anything but.

A group of doctors and nurses arrived. I feared it might have been the moment of truth. The lead doctor examined the large lump on the right side of my head and forehead, where the helmet had protected me and split in the impact. He carefully prodded around my right collarbone, which I felt quite obviously was broken. I told him my hips and lower back were emitting extraordinarily high levels of pain and said I was most concerned that I could not seem to move my legs. He recorded my symptoms and description of the road impact and the accident before looking at my legs, back or hips.

I was lifted up onto the board above the group to have my spine examined by the doctor. He pressed one vertebrae at a time from my neck to hips. It felt quite precarious being held off the floor and above the trolley by a team of doctors and nurses. He asked me to tell him what I could feel and proceeded to prod each vertebrae in turn. When he reached my lower back I felt a sudden excruciating sharp wave of pain, replicated all the way to his final press to conclude the examination. The anticipation of each prod was awful, bringing familiar waves of pain back to the fore as my hips and back were checked. This time the pain medication did not provide quite the protection I had hoped for.

I was put down and left in the A&E cubicle with my thoughts. I could hear the muffled conversation between the ambulance team and again tried to unsuccessfully divert my thoughts about the implications of a spinal injury. Again and again the constant fear prompted by my inability to use or feel my legs kept returning.

Tania arrived. She did well to keep the tone light given the situation. She told me the man who had put me in hospital had been driving off oblivious to the damage he had caused and explained that she had to shout for him to stop his car. She said the driver, who was in his mid eighties, had been interviewed by the police. She too had given an accident report to officers, one of whom had driven her to the hospital.

As a medical professional herself, I was confident she had also given a concise report to the doctors who were in the process of assessing and diagnosing my injuries. We deliberately avoided discussing or speculating what the injuries might be.

Vital information for emergency services:

1. What happened and whether you saw it

2. The estimated speed of vehicles involved

3. How much time has passed since the accident happened

4. Whether the patient has been conscious since the accident, including lapses into unconsciousness

5. Have they been talking sensibly or confused and moaning

6. Have there been any fits for seizures

7. A top-to-toe summary of injuries

8. What you have done to treat any injuries

9. Whether the patient has been moving their arms and legs

Kate McCombe, *consultant anaesthetist, and* **Kelvin Wright**, *consultant in Emergency Medicine and Critical Care, Frimley Park Hospital, Surrey.*

It felt surreal that life could change so quickly as a result of someone else's careless actions. We avoided talking about the injuries. She reassured me that she was ok, and I would be too now that I was in the hospital.

Then I was taken for X-rays, which took some time, before being slid into a CT machine for a full scan. At every move there was the horrible feeling of bones grinding against each other, which triggered a fresh burst of fear over my continued failure to engage with my legs or move properly.

I was starting to feel quite exhausted and fell asleep inside the CT machine despite the rhythmical mechanical noise and claustrophobic environment. The sharp sheet tug back on to the trolley was painful and surprising. It had been a lengthy process, and I had lost track of what time of day it was. I wondered if it was the pain medication or trauma of the accident that was making me feel so tired and unable to stay awake.

Once I was taken back to the A&E ward, Tania was waiting for me with a police officer. A nurse settled me in, and the police officer asked whether I would be prepared to answer some questions about the accident. It didn't start well when he said it looked like I had taken a 'little tumble' from my bike. His sense of humour and approach was not lost on me, lying in A&E with an oxygen mask on, hooked up to a number of flashing monitors. I felt as though I should have been sat with a plaster on my knee instead.

Tania helpfully lifted and lowered the oxygen mask as I responded to the officer's questions. I was amazed at the details that I could remember, as though the situation presented itself in slow motion. I acknowledged that I might not have survived the double impact and injuries had I not opted for a race-honed, emergency braking technique in order to avoid going into or over the driver's vehicle. I had been focused on actions that avoided a double impact: the driver's car and into oncoming traffic, or the driver's car and road.

'Survival mechanisms are so strong in an emergency situation, provoking what would usually be unusual, unrealistic reactions or movement in order to survive.'

Tania Cotton
Health in Motion founder, movement analyst, British chartered physiotherapist

It was clear that Tania had only just avoided being taken out by the driver herself or riding into me as I hit the road, and she had been riding at least 10 bike lengths behind me. The police officer had noted my speed at 30 mph. Many months later when I downloaded the Garmin bike computer file, I saw from the GPS data that my bike was travelling at approximately 38 to 40 kph when the car pulled in front of me. I was very lucky to have been able to avoid him and his car with just 3 to 5 metres to react with.

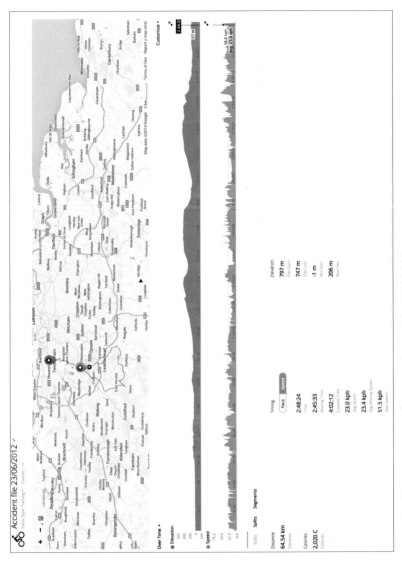

Garmin ride file – see connect.garmin.com/modern/activity/273554750

I was relieved when the police officer left, slightly bemused by his approach and very grateful when my regular cycling buddy Kerrie arrived with Tania and a small cup of water. Answering all of the questions had left me exhausted, and I was feeling increasingly dehydrated as the afternoon wore on. There were a few tears as I greeted Kerrie from the hospital bed. We would normally have been cycling together except she had been racing this weekend. We chatted about her performance, which was a welcome change of subject, while waiting for the results of the tests.

A doctor arrived. He informed me that I had what was regarded as serious injuries. These were later described in the hospital report as 'life-changing'. The test results confirmed a broken right clavicle, along with a broken pelvis and sacrum. I digested the information. He had made no mention of my spine or spinal damage. That was good news, surely?

I didn't fully understand the implications of a broken pelvis or sacrum or why it would mean my legs appeared not to be working properly. The doctor explained that fracturing the pelvis completely was serious. Both the inferior and superior pubic rami were broken through, and the diagonally opposite sacrum at the base of my spine on the left side was fractured as a result. These injuries were apparently typical of a high-impact fall or impact.

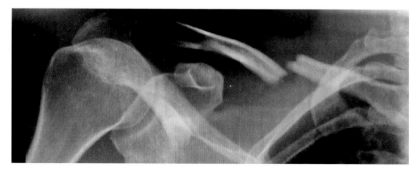

Right clavicle fracture

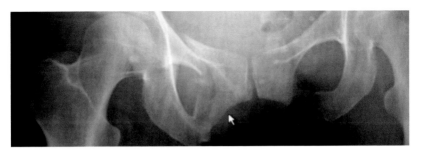

Superior and inferior fracture pelvis, right side

On Monday he said a consultant team would be in a position to advise the best course of treatment for my injuries and would be able to tell me whether I would need an operation on my pelvis. He left after explaining I would need a further X-ray on my lower back before being moved to a room on the ward overnight.

After a few goodbyes and hugs, Kerrie and Tania left, with a bag containing all of my kit and a few personal items. Now I knew what I was dealing with, I felt overwhelmed, and another wave of emotion hit me, leaving me exhausted.

I really wanted to speak to my parents, but they lived in Australia and I realised it was the early hours of the morning there. I didn't want to worry them. I suddenly hoped I might wake up and find that I had in fact been in a dream all along, a really bad one.

I was soon wheeled away to a room on the ward after being X-rayed again. There was a short wait and thankfully the nurse wheeling me down corridors and in the lift was interested in triathlon and running, so we chatted as we went. The nurse explained that I would be taken to a separate room on the 'hip' ward due to being the youngest patient, meaning it would be quieter and likely to expedite my rest and therefore recovery. I was finding it difficult to process this information in context, fighting off a strong desire to sleep.

I could hear a range of noises, beeps, moans and crying out coming from the ward where most of the patients were elderly. I was quite grateful when I was wheeled into a small room and settled into a separate, quieter space.

Once the A&E nurse left and I had been checked for the evening, I had a few small sips of water. I recognised it was quite late in the day and how readily I wanted to sleep. The routine noises of a busy hospital ward, regular buzzing, distant voices and discomfort of lying on my back all paled into insignificance as I closed my eyes on the most turbulent day of my life so far. I felt extremely lucky to be alive.

Coping strategies while you wait for diagnosis of injuries:

Understand that your range of skills and developed racing strategies may have saved your life. Being able to respond rather than react adversely to intensely provoking situations can make the difference between surviving serious injuries or a fatal accident.

Reflect on the subconscious process you may have used in the moments before the impact in reaction to circumstances. Fractions of a second will have provided you with options for you to immediately decide the best course of action.

Explain what you remember of the accident to your friends or family once your condition is stable and you are no longer in tremendous amounts of pain. Being able to synthesise the information and sensory clues, particularly the visual aspects to someone, helps to recall details and facts very likely to be important in recording your accident clearly.

Discuss the scene from your friend or training companion's perspective, too. Have them make notes on anything you may wish to check later, such as your bike computer for data.

Acknowledge and draw strength from how you reacted under pressure. Being living proof of this personal asset is a positive outcome to focus on throughout the difficult times ahead and learn from the experience.

'Feel the fear and focus on the positives.'

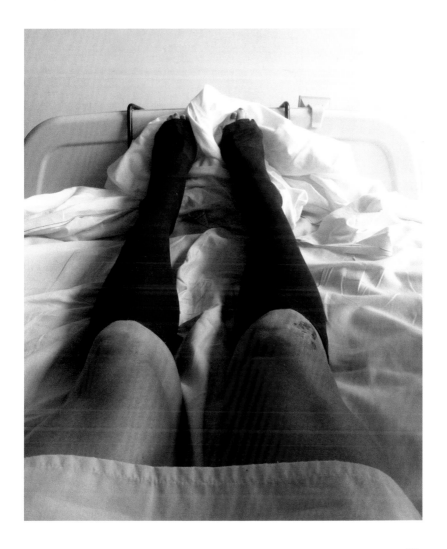

CHAPTER 3:
LIFE-CHANGING INJURIES

Biggest achievement: Moving toes 1 cm

Top speed: 0 kph
Elevation gain: 0 m
Distance: 0 m

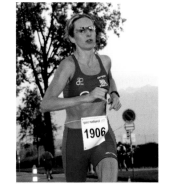

6 am Sunday 24 June 2012

I was running, racing and feeling the ground move swiftly beneath my feet. I received a shout from one of my supporters that I was at least two minutes up the road on my competitors. The feedback didn't influence me to slow my pace or rhythm one little bit; if anything it spurred me on to extend the gap further.

Months of physical preparation and powerful visualisation techniques had brought me to this point: racing at the ITU World Championships (2006) in Lausanne, Switzerland and turning in the best possible performance I could deliver as an age group athlete.

Now it was just me, the course, conditions, the clock and what I could do across the three disciplines of swim, bike and run.

I could feel myself almost choking with the effort and emotion of delivering a lifetime best performance. I tried again to take a deep breath and suddenly felt my body radiating with pain.

While racing I hadn't expected such twisting, sharp pains coming from my back, hips, shoulder, fingertips, neck and head. Something was seriously wrong.

Then suddenly I felt consciously aware that I appeared to be in a hospital bed hooked up to alien medical equipment, a sling on my right arm unable to move properly. How could this be? Had I taken a fall during a race? Perhaps at the World Championships? It was the wrong race; the timescale didn't make sense to me on any level.

My mind scrambled to make sense of the new waking reality I was faced with, but suddenly the memory focused sharply into view. It had been a training accident. The road came up to meet me as I flew helplessly through the air attached to my race bike, my brain providing the horrifying replay on command.

I closed my eyes again and felt tears streaming down my face. The shock of waking up to find it really had happened made me feel sick.

I distracted myself with the present, starting a methodical head-to-toe assessment. My face and the right side of my head felt raw, bruised and painful; a lump had grown under my hairline where the helmet had cracked in two.

I carefully touched along the length of the lump from my forehead along the side of my head. No wonder I had a headache! My right shoulder ached with the dull throb of the collarbone fractured halfway along its length.

Gently feeling along the swelling of the right shoulder with my left hand revealed the whole area was distended and bruised. The fingertips on my left hand were raw because of the missing flesh. The back of my right shoulder also felt like it was stuck to the bedsheets. This was the rawness of road rash, I presumed.

I shifted the sling a little to take some of the weight off the shoulder and then attempted to shuffle up the bed a little more into a sitting position using my left arm to support me. This was a bad idea. Even the smallest movement of my upper body set off a chain reaction of pain. My lower back felt strange, heavy and tingled farther down where it joined my hips, which sat heavily on the mattress.

I decided to experiment with moving my legs one at a time to relieve some of the numbness. I managed to persuade my left knee into a tiny amount of flexion, but it seemed to take ages and required significant levels of concentration.

I tried the same strategy with the right leg, but it was unresponsive. I gritted my teeth and resolved to move it even a millimetre. I was shocked to find the neuromuscular connection between mental will and movement was not working.

I quickly revised my expectations and tried instead to move my toes. Relief. I managed a wiggle on both sides, although it was a little slower going on the right. It felt painfully nice to stretch my toes and flex my feet even the tiniest amount under the sheet and light hospital blanket. I noticed the range improved accordingly. It was a positive sign, which kept me occupied for many minutes.

A nurse appeared and carried out the early morning checks on blood pressure, heart rate and temperature. She noted my heart rate was 'low' at 46 beats per minute (bpm), which was, apparently, a concern. If it was a worry to her, it wasn't to me. I had seen it at 42 bpm when measuring it first thing in the morning at peak racing condition. After being assessed by a senior nurse and answering her questions about performing a significant amount of exercise on a regular basis, she was satisfied 46 bpm was acceptable due to the amount of exercise I was used to doing.

I could hear activity outside the room. I recognised the smell of breakfast and realised morning rounds were in full swing. The nurse said I would soon be seen by the doctors and gave me a range of painkillers to take with some water.

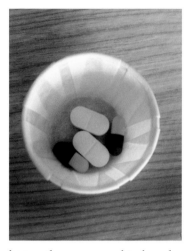

One of four daily doses of analgesics tramadol and paracetemol

Two nurses came in with fresh bed linen and a new gown. After a bed wash of the non-broken bits of my body, it took only a few minutes to remove and replace the gown and manoeuvre the ties under my back and shoulders. The efficiency with which they whipped the damp sheet out from underneath me was reassuringly painless. To my horror there appeared to be a large amount of blood on the sheet, which I had been unaware of. This was quite normal for pelvic fractures I was told. After the nurses were finished, I closed my eyes.

When I opened them again, five doctors were crowding into the room by the foot of my bed. The lead consultant introduced himself and his colleagues before proceeding to rattle through a list of my injuries: broken right clavicle, broken left sacrum and a compression fracture of the pelvis, meaning both inferior and superior pubic rami were broken. Translated into English, that meant my pelvis was completely shattered, and my collarbone had snapped in two.

Then he let me have it. He told me my injuries were very serious due to the speed at which they had occurred. It was unlikely I would be able to run again. One of his colleagues added that my marathon running days were over. As they dropped this information all very matter-of-fact, they could have no idea of the impact it was having on someone who had been born for endurance sport. At this point all I wanted to know was whether I would be able to walk again. The far-reaching implications had not sunk in at all. Surely they had skipped over the obvious advice?

They told me there would be no food until Monday when my scans and X-rays would have been assessed and the specialist doctors had decided whether they needed to operate or not. I was left in silence, stunned by the implications of their words and confused by the lack of clarity over my future.

Then the leading consultant took me completely by surprise. 'So just how good a triathlete are you then?'

I answered him briefly, summarising the past decade competing as a world-class age group (amateur) athlete, former two-time world and European champion at Olympic/standard distance triathlon.

I explained that for the past three years I had been racing in the pro ranks at Ironman® distance – sponsored by a bike company – producing seven top 10 finishes and earning prize money whilst working full-time running my coaching business.

I paused. It suddenly felt a bit embarrassing to be discussing my athletic CV with a team of doctors, especially when my livelihood was looking more than a little under threat.

I asked the doctor whether he had competed in triathlons. He answered briefly that he had and wanted to know my personal best over Olympic distance. '2:09,' I replied. That ended the conversation.

One of the junior doctors asked me whether I would like to see the X-rays and offered to capture a picture on my battered and bent phone for me to see, which I handed over. She soon returned with the image after the team had left and explained the fractures of my pelvis to me in more depth. I was very grateful for her time. When she left, the confusion and mixed feelings set in.

Recommended medical protocol for injury assessment:

1. Listen – fundamental. If the patient has back pain, it needs to be checked. Athletes particularly have greater awareness of their bodies and pain thresholds.

2. Top-to-toe check using scans, X-rays and physical observation.

3. History of what happened and patient medical health to discover biggest clues.

4. Download information from all sources then apply expertise, not rushing to diagnose or assess patient condition until all facts are known or available.

5. Patient empowerment – never make decisions for the patient. Present the options. For an athlete function and movement range are paramount if they are to resume their sport eventually.

Tania Cotton, *Health in Motion founder, movement analyst, British chartered physiotherapist*

It was late morning, and I realised it was probably an ideal time to call my parents in Australia. I had wanted to call them before but the time difference meant it was not possible. It's bad enough making the call lying broken in hospital explaining you have been involved in a bike crash caused by a car without breaking the news at 1 am.

I figured they would be about to settle down on the sofa after a busy weekend and Sunday roast dinner. It seemed like the right time. I dialled their home number from my mobile. When my father answered, I explained briefly where I was and what had happened. I heard the shock in his voice and reassured him that I was ok before speaking to my mother.

It's one of the most difficult phone calls I have ever had with my mum, and just hearing her voice left me struggling to speak for a few minutes. She asked me if they needed to come over (I had never needed her so much), but I told her to wait until I knew what my treatment would be.

Upset and exhausted, I fell asleep for a few hours and consoled myself that at least my pain levels were being managed by a regular four-hour intake of medication and that I didn't have to move. It felt good to just stop and rest.

It was all I wanted to do most of that day. I had never been so incredibly overwhelmed with tiredness; the levels simply didn't compare with Ironman®- or marathon-induced fatigue for weeks after the many gruelling endurance or multisport events I had done over the years.

I had no appetite for food, and my dehydration was finally under control, so it was all about sleep.

Side effects of analgesics:

Tramadol

» Dizziness

» Nausea and vomiting

» Constipation

» Drowsiness

» Headache

Patients may experience less commonly:

>> Agitation

>> Anxiety

>> Emotional lability

>> Euphoria

>> Disordered sleep

>> Itchiness

Paracetamol

>> Very rare in prescribed doses

Ibuprofen

>> Nausea

>> Indigestion

>> 10-20% of asthmatics find their asthma is exacerbated

Less commonly experienced, in severe cases:

>> Stomach ulceration and bleeding

Kate McCombe, *consultant anaesthetist, Frimley Park Hospital, Surrey*

My life was about as physical as you could get. It wasn't just that I was a pro endurance athlete, I was also a coach with a successful business painstakingly built up over many years. Starting my own business had been a big risk and a leap of faith. It's not easy to give up the regular pay, pension and perks of the 9-5 job.

When I wasn't training, I was training others. I was walking the poolside, assessing stroke, gait and revolutions. I was demonstrating. I was animated. And I had a strong team of paying athletes on my books. In short nothing in my life was done with ease while lying on a bed with only one hand free to operate a mobile phone. That was not my life. It was not even close.

That said, thankfully my thumb was still in good enough shape for the iPhone swipe, so I checked for messages and emails. I saw, ruefully, that my 7 am Sunday morning swim workshop had been cancelled by my PA. She was on the case of other coaching activities that would need to be scrapped.

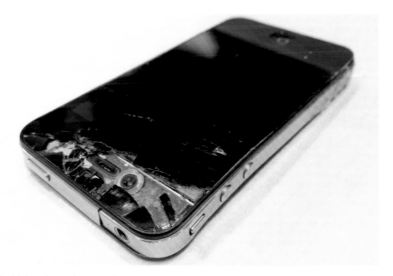

Survived iPhone in rear jersey pocket

A few of my coached athletes and good friends had offered to help when they heard I had been hit, so I set about arranging cover for some of my squad sessions that week and making alternative arrangements for the athletes.

Sorting out my short-term commitments meant I could put off thinking about the long-term impact of my injuries. All I had to concentrate on was juggling the phone with one arm as I ploughed on with business as (un)usual.

My friends drew up a visiting rota so that I would have a regular stream of visitors every day. That evening I had recounted the accident a number of times. Each time I came back to the underlying question about the driver's mistake.

I felt anger and the full implications of having let my private health insurance lapse for the first time in my life earlier that month. Why didn't the driver bother to look to his right before driving out of the side road and across the right of way? How could he be so careless with a life? What if he had looked? What if? What if?

What you want from your friends during their hospital visits:

DO

1. Get friends and family to organise a visiting rota – little and often to help keep spirits up and not overwhelm.

2. Bring food – hospital food really is as bad as everyone says, and good nutrition is the key to recovery.

3. Offer to help, including arrangements for things around the home as well as chasing down medical staff.

4. Get them to bring in the home comforts – slippers, pyjamas, underwear, facewash, moisturiser and shampoo. There's nothing better for making you feel human.

DON'T

1. Outstay your welcome – keep the visits to 30 minutes, or you will exhaust the patient.

2. Pass out. In the event of hearing the details of the injuries try not to faint. The nurses have enough to do. (Yes, my friend/s, you will remain nameless!)

3. Talk about 'life before the accident' or try to make light of it by saying 'you'll be racing again soon'. Positive is one thing, ridiculous statements are another.

4. Bring children. Children are lovely, but they are noisy and easily bored in a hospital room. Not ideal for recuperating adults.

How tired?

Extremely high fatigue levels are one of the most significant side effects to serious injury recovery that an active person finds difficult to understand and cope with.

Go beyond listening to your body's needs, and rest as regularly as you need in immediate days after a major trauma. This will greatly assist your recovery process.

'Your body's ability to heal is far greater than anything you have been led to believe.'

CHAPTER 4:
HOSPITAL FOOD

Biggest achievement: Being able to walk with support, under careful supervision

Top speed: 0.1 kph
Elevation gain: 1 m from floor to hospital bed
Distance: 10 m

Monday 25 June 2012 – millimetres of movement

The rhythm and noise of buzzers, beeps, murmured voices, activity and rising pain levels brought me out of sleep the next morning.

After being checked on by the nurse and given my morning pain medication, I preoccupied myself with what had become my routine head-to-toe check. I surveyed my tanned, toned but seemingly useless legs and noted a slight improvement in the way I could move my toes.

The effort of focusing on lifting any part of either leg from the bed was immense. Everything had to be initiated through the hips and my core, which seemingly were not in communication with each other. In contrast to the effort and focus, the range of movement was minimal. I managed to gently tighten and relax my quads, which helped release some of the numbness caused by lying on my backside for hours.

My left hamstring threatened to cramp, and I was quickly reminded the extreme pain levels were still there. I switched my attention to my lower back and shoulders, trying to slightly shift position in the bed to remove some of the pressure and discomfort from my hips.

A weird tingling sensation emanated from my right side, presumably where my back and hips had met the road, cushioned only by my mobile phone. Judging by its bent and battered state, I considered the damage and imprint that I could feel in the soft tissue of my lower back and hip. My right shoulder seemed hot and distended, and the sling supporting it felt heavy with the weight of the arm.

The lump on my head still felt sore, and the grazes on my fingers and hand were raw. A massive bruise had developed on most of my left arm, from the cannula insertion attempts on the roadside at the accident site.

I longed for a proper shower and to wash my face and hair. An overwhelming desire to cleanse the road grime and sweaty anxiety away dominated my thoughts, and I contemplated if I could make the bathroom.

The door was only a metre or two from my bed. What, I wondered, would happen if I tried to gently lower myself out of bed? Would I be able to support myself and stand upright? Or would this result in my legs crumbling and a painful fall onto a very hard-looking surface? I had temporarily forgotten that the combination of multiple injuries meant I had lost mobility and ability to swing both legs out of bed and standing on my own two feet.

In the end I calculated the move was high risk, and I stayed where I was safely corralled in the hospital bed. It dawned on me that I was completely reliant on those around me to help with every aspect of day-to-day life. I had lost all of my independence and ability to look after myself, something I had taken for granted all my adult life. Being hooked up to a catheter meant no trips to the bathroom were necessary, and an IV drip kept me hydrated.

Later that morning the team of doctors appeared on their rounds. They had come to deliver their decision about treatment of my injuries. Having consulted with the specialist consultant for pelvic injuries it had been decided conservative treatment was the best option. That meant no operation.

Instead I would be encouraged to start standing up and bearing weight as soon as possible to encourage the pelvic fractures to mend. I was surprised because the seriousness of the injuries had been explained to me to indicate an operation would be necessary.

As they filed out, I was left feeling vulnerable and worried about the proposed course of treatment. It was hard not to think about questions concerning how well the fractures would mend by themselves.

I managed to respond to some emails on my phone and make necessary arrangements for squad training to proceed that evening in my absence. I feared that years of work, long hours, creating a diverse coaching business, building my client base and honing coaching methods and systems would start to unravel pretty quickly if I were unable to coach, compete and train with my athletes. The prospect of losing my livelihood began to sink in.

Searching for the bright side – and there was one – what I did take from the doctors' visit was that I could eat again. My lack of appetite since Saturday afternoon had astonished me. I had never experienced a three-day period where my stomach hadn't reminded me to fuel for multiple daily training sessions.

The problem was when lunch appeared, I wasn't overly enthusiastic about the processed food on offer. I normally cooked meals from scratch with fresh ingredients. Hospital food could not get further away from my normal diet – it looked like it had been created in a laboratory, not a kitchen. My lack of appetite and low energy meant I needed an abundance of fresh, antioxidant-rich foods to support the full-scale repair process. It wasn't going to be found on the hospital menu!

A young physiotherapist visited me mid-afternoon to complete an assessment of my injuries, range of movement and mobility. She informed me that I was scheduled for 'conservative treatment' of my multiple fractures to the right side of my pelvis and left sacrum, meaning that I would be aiming to weight bear through my hips and pelvis as soon as possible.

Alarm bells: How would this be possible when everything felt broken and disconnected through the middle? The assessment showed I could move my right leg a little more than a few millimetres by myself. The left leg was a little more able to interpret messages from my brain, to lift and bend at the knee, pull my toes and feet towards my shin and stretch and push the leg away. She encouraged me to practise a basic set of movement exercises a few more times during the remainder of the day.

I spent the day resting and dozing on and off with the combination of tramadol, ibuprofen and paracetamol keeping pain levels just about manageable. Two of my close friends and athletes Tarek and Josh visited me later in the afternoon. They brought proper food. Josh had even smuggled in some flowers for me, which were definitely not allowed!

The highlight of my evening was a wonderful photo taken of the swim squad as they completed their cool-down, all holding up the letters to make up a 'get well Coach Fi' sign between them. I received the text just as I was dozing off for the evening, and it helped me feel better about all of the support needed to keep key activities going in my absence.

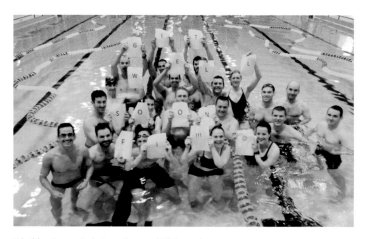

Triathlon Europe SwimSmooth squad, Richmond

Tuesday 26 June 2012 – 'Conservative treatment'

The next morning I woke early to the all-over, and by now familiar, sensation of bones aching. Ouch. I wondered if I would ever get used to sleeping on my back, with my right arm in a sling. After my pain medication was delivered with some water by the nurse and my vital signs checked, I started my day with a hot water and green tea, grateful for supplies brought in the previous day.

I started on my leg exercises and my morning head-to-toe body check. My right leg was still very reluctant to move more than the few millimetres it had managed the day before, but with determination to repeat the lifting and lowering of my knees and stretching through my feet and ankles, the pain barrier was successfully challenged and overcome.

It was tiring to push through the pain from multiple injury sites; however, I could see progress with the left leg and hoped some of this positivity would transfer over to the more 'broken' side. My lower back was extremely painful and disconnected if I tried to shift my weight up the bed, using the support of my good arm.

This morning's discovery by the nurses was the rectangular imprint of my iPhone above my right hip on my side and lower back. I couldn't see it, but could feel the pain when the raised, bruised skin was gently washed. I could also see just how much damage had been done to my left arm with the numerous unsuccessful cannula attempts at the accident scene.

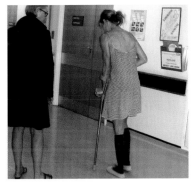

First walking steps under careful supervision of friend Susan

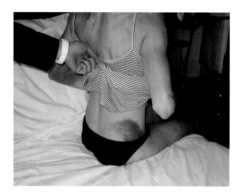

One of the many impact sites with the road, cushioned by iPhone

Checking in with work and emails, I was extremely relieved to discover my mum would be making the long flight from Sydney within the next few days to help with my care once I left hospital.

12:00 Physiotherapy

After I had received late-morning pain medication, it was time for physiotherapy, starting with a round of questioning about the accident, what I did for a living and my level of fitness.

A recap on yesterday's exercises showed a little improvement in flexion through the knee, particularly on the left side. It seemed as though my progress was expected to be rapid to a weight-bearing stage. I had confidence that if it was physically possible then my body would be able to achieve it. I had rarely had any cause to doubt what my body was capable of, in any training or hundreds of events I had raced in the past decade.

The reality of movement, however, seemed to suggest otherwise, and I hit off-the-scale pain levels within minutes. The physio's main objective was for me to lift my knees and move my legs a little more than the previous day. Simple right?

My right leg was extraordinarily painful to move millimetres, the hip flexor and adductor connecting to my hip were unable to support the heavy limb. However, the left leg demonstrated improved range and comparatively less pain.

Pain came from all around the hips and my lower back as we worked through the simplest of exercises to move my feet centimetre by centimetre from side to side and lifting or bending the knees a few centimetres from the bed. The concentration levels required were immense, given the small movement produced.

Still progress is progress – and there was some. I could move a few more millimetres each time I tried. Gaining respite from the pain became a reward for pushing through painful range of movement. It felt strangely satisfying, like a tough training session without the associated endorphins.

'Focus on what you can do, not what you can't. Remain positive by doing what you can do in the moment.'

Dave Scott, *Six-time Ironman® Triathlon World Championship winner*

The physiotherapy session only lasted 10 to 15 minutes, but I felt exhausted enough to nap until lunch arrived.

14:00

After a dose of liquid morphine I agreed to another physiotherapy session and was given the task of moving down the bed. My objective for the afternoon was reach the side and to stand up with assistance.

I began the slow, painful process using my left arm to push, lift and manoeuvre myself millimetre by millimetre down and along the bed, gritting my teeth as I went. She suggested if it hurt too much then more morphine was the solution. I was not convinced.

As I reached the side of the bed I was feeling sick from all the effort. I eased my legs over the edge. The pain was excruciating as my legs plunged towards the floor, and there was a crunching as my middle seemed to move, disconnected. My view of the room narrowed in tunnel vision, and my temperature shot up.

Poor Kerrie, who had arrived for a visit and ended up watching my progress, could cope no longer. She found it impossible to watch and put her head in her hands before leaving the room. She later confessed the audible sound of my injuries as I moved off the bed had been too much.

The physio encouraged me to try to lower my feet to touch the floor, as I sat attempting to compose myself on the edge of the bed, supporting my upper body with my left arm. I felt as though I would be sick or pass out at any moment.

After a pause, breathing deeply, I overcame the overwhelming sensation, and the pain levels subsided a little. I wanted to get a grip on being able to perform this very simple task. It was time to try again. My left foot made contact with the floor, followed gingerly by my right. After a few attempts I managed to stand up supported by the physio.

Extreme nausea and dizziness was accompanied by another awful bone-crunching sound. Standing and wobbling on both feet holding on to the physio felt unlike anything I had ever experienced before. She asked me to try and lift one leg forward and then the other.

Excruciating cramps set off around my hips, glutes, hamstrings and lower back as I attempted to shift weight to one foot while I moved the other a tiny centimetre forward. The left foot moved a little, but it took three attempts to drag the foot along the floor a centimetre. I could not lift the right foot from the floor at all.

I sank gratefully back onto the bed, took a deep breath and composed myself in small victory. I had just managed to stand up on my legs!

When the physio left and Kerrie returned, we discussed what I had just managed to do. Despite incredibly high pain levels, it was clear that I was going to be able to walk again, with focus and determination.

Exhausted and elated, I even found a little more enthusiasm for my dinner when it arrived.

Wednesday 27 June 2012 – The 'marathon' walk

I started the day with a breakfast of the familiar yellow and green pills (tramadol and ibuprofen) some nuts and seeds from supplies brought in by friends, yoghurt and green tea. My morning physio visit involved checking in to see how my morning exercises were going and an assessment for a walking frame.

She left hurriedly, explaining she wanted me to have some morphine administered before she returned for our session around midday. The doctor's round was brief, almost like my care had been pigeon-holed into conservative which was a convenient and time-effective solution for them.

I asked about the neck and back X-ray as had been suggested and was informed that just my pelvis would be X-rayed every week for three weeks to discuss with the specialists. I was told the clavicle would heal itself, but it was clear to me the bones were nearly 2 centimetres apart, and I couldn't see how that would be possible. I had previously fractured my left clavicle falling from a racehorse and that had mended without surgery, but the bones had still been in alignment. It was clear even at this early stage I was going to require a second opinion.

I managed to carry out some work again, by way of emails on my phone. My morning was made with the positive news and confirmation from my parents that my mum was on her way from Sydney to London. This filled me with confidence, happiness and hope. Mum being a real 'foodie' meant an added bonus that my appetite might be coaxed back into operation.

12:00 Physiotherapy

The physio appeared with a tall walking frame on wheels. It looked a cumbersome bit of equipment, but I was keen to see whether I could use it. Could I possibly take some steps today?

I was helped to stand and transfer my weight to the walking frame, which was steadied by the physio. Standing, I waited until the horrible associated crunching and pain through my pelvis had stopped making me feel sick and dizzy.

I was about to learn to walk again. 'Begin with the left leg', I thought as I tried to lift it from the floor. It was very reluctant to move, and I opted instead to drag it a few centimetres. I could lift most of the foot, except the big toe, away from the floor, but to fully support it in midair was a significant challenge.

It was time to try the other side. However, the cramps setting off in muscle groups all around the pelvis and lower back were debilitating.

I had to stop, try to balance, stand, lean on the frame and allow this intolerable cramping to die down. It took a few minutes before I could control the pain sufficiently to switch focus to the right foot and leg. The objective to move the leg seemed blocked between brain and muscles

I had to really focus to achieve the tiniest movement. Though incredibly painfully, I managed to shuffle the foot with the slightest heel lift a few millimetres forward. I realised I was sweating with the effort.

Another focused few minutes, and I had the left foot co-operating, taking another step and dragging the toe a few more centimetres. The cramping of my glute and hamstring on the left side was off the scale compared with anything I had ever experienced in training or a race. I stopped again to allow the spasms to stop before trying the right leg again.

Another shuffle with the foot barely leaving the floor, apart from the heel. It was incredible, I was moving forward!

Continued attempts to push through the pain barrier with each leg movement were rewarded with tiny shuffling steps absorbed by a hunched body over the walking frame. I reached the door of my room, nearly four metres away from the bed where I had started and stopped to rest.

I felt as though I had run a marathon. It had taken the best part of 20 minutes – the same amount of time it would have taken me to run 5 kilometres – and do a series of stretches and take a drink afterwards (my personal best over 5k was 16.58 min).

The physio advised how I was to turn around safely. There was not much space to manoeuvre myself and the frame to make my way back to the bed. I opted to turn towards my less mobile side, the right, so the left leg could take the proportionately larger and longer steps required to make a 180-degree turn.

Millimetres at a time I slowly angled my steps around, noticing that my lower back around the sacrum fracture constantly spasmed with any lateral movement. The return journey back to the bed took many minutes; however, I could feel that some improvement in the frequency of steps had been made, although the pain was no less.

I was helped back into bed. It was amazing to consider how much more tiring the process of moving an injured body just four days after a serious accident was compared with the rigours of a day-long physical event racing an Ironman® triathlon. Never after those seven occasions during a 10-hour race had I ever felt as battered and totally worn out as I did that afternoon.

Tips to maximise the early rehabilitation process back to functional movement:

>> Record your progress.

>> Note up to 3 short-term goals.

>> Focus on the present; don't get too far ahead of yourself.

>> It's ok to feel stretched and challenged during initial rehabilitation.

>> Aim to replicate functional movement.

>> Use pain medication to help you establish weight-bearing movement under supervision.

>> Celebrate every success, no matter how incremental.

» Review progress towards goals; set new objectives.

» Recognise improvement and consistency in achievements.

» Walk before you try to run!

My afternoon visitor Adam, the masters swim coach from Teddington Swimming Club, was a wonderful inspiration and support. He was a very talented swimmer and always able to get the best out of those he coached with softly spoken, perfectly timed encouragement. He was exactly who I needed to see before my evening round of physiotherapy.

We discussed the accident, the training sessions I was missing this week and how my squads were going to be covered in my absence. He offered any help I might need and reassured me that I would be able to recover from the injuries I had, using the skills and attitude of a champion athlete.

It was really positive to envisage being at a stage of rehab in the open air pool at Hampton, where I regularly trained with the masters. This idyllic thought of a heated outdoor pool, familiar environment, sun and a routine I was already missing a lot meant the world to me. I looked forward to being able to draw on Adam's offer of support when I was ready to start swimming again. It seemed a long way off from where I lay in the hospital bed that afternoon.

15:00

Having had my usual four-hour pain medication, I was keen to try the afternoon walk without a dose of liquid morphine to try and limit the nausea and dizziness. I wondered if it was better to deal with the 'real' situation of the pain.

While it felt like a breakthrough to be up on my feet taking tiny steps, I also had doubts that I needed to be doing so much, so soon. I usually listened to the high levels of fatigue, but I felt I should attempt a second walk that day and so prepared myself.

As I moved I realised I was thinking through the process of how to perform movements which had been unconsciously made thousands of times in my life before. I grasped the walking frame and committed to the painful process of standing up and the consequences that would follow. The wave of nausea came and went after the initial energy rush and audible movement within the injury sites.

I focused on the padded top of the frame as the dizziness dissolved, resting some of my weight on the left arm and elbow. This time I was able to cover more distance, and I steadily inched my way out of the room into the main corridor opposite all the activity of the central nurse station.

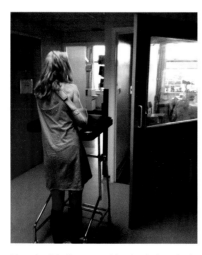

First 'walking' steps with the help of the walking frame

It felt like a huge achievement to be outside the security and safety of my room. My right leg continued to be the most difficult to move, requiring specific focus to shift my weight to the left and gritting resolve to activate the very painful hip flexor and opposite glute.

My slow and painful shuffle back towards my bed culminated in double the distance I had covered earlier in the afternoon and felt an amazing achievement.

I started to inwardly refer to my physio as the 'physio-terrorist'. Her priority was clearly to get me mobile and on my way out of hospital as soon as possible.

As a coach and athlete, I found it seemed alien to use medication to mask symptoms of pain in order to achieve as much movement as possible. I really wasn't keen on taking morphine on a regular basis, along with the regular combination of medication I was taking all day long to manage pain levels when at rest.

The session ended with me being encouraged to get my legs back into the bed by myself. I was informed that I would progress to crutches as soon as possible. With pain levels just about manageable I was not keen to risk a fall and further injuring myself having only just started to take my first tiny, toe-dragging steps.

Thursday 28 June 2012

After a troubled night sweating, suffering from accident flashbacks and unmanageable pain, I woke feeling like I had not slept at all. I raised my concerns about the shoulder perhaps not healing conservatively during the doctor's rounds. It too was disturbed by the amount of activity the day before when my overwhelming desire was to rest and let the pain levels become manageable.

11:45 Physiotherapy

My morning physio with a different therapist seemed way too early as my body didn't feel rested or recovered from the previous day. However, I did feel motivated to use the walking frame and repeat another attempt at a 'walk' out into the corridor again.

The challenge to shuffle centimetres at a time and ignore the pain levels, nausea and light headedness was starting to pay off. I could feel more response in both legs, although I still struggled to lift either leg and foot fully off the floor.

Dragging by the toe was functional to a point, but the physio said I should try to lift the leg and swing it forward rather than allow it to slide the few centimetres at a time. Saying it was simple; doing it not so.

The sense of the hip flexor joining into something unstable or bone that was moving didn't help my efforts to push beyond what my body could manage.

I was used to operating at my physical limits, but it also meant I knew well when broken areas just could not function in the normal way. Today's 'objective' soon became clear. The new therapist was keen to have me walk with the frame to the bathroom to test whether I could use the facilities and walk back out again. The most difficult issue was fitting myself and the walking frame into the confined space and safely moving around. I didn't want to knock myself against anything in the small space or fall down. I met the challenge.

I had to make a few calls to cancel appointments planned for that week and next and also speak with Surrey police for an update on the accident report and driver's details. Just an hour of work after the rigours of the morning induced an overwhelming need to close my eyes and rest.

Practicalities of dealing with challenges of time in hospital:

With a little help from your friends and family, the following strategies provide helpful solutions

>> Making arrangements for responsibilities at home – pets or other family

>> Managing anxieties around work, assisting with updates on timescales

>> Understanding the impact of injuries on wider aspects of life in context, not in isolation

>> Reassuring and helping to find solutions to practical issues Following up medical advice or recommendations

>> Sourcing specific kit or aids

Tania Cotton, *Health in Motion founder, movement analyst, British chartered physiotherapist*

Kerrie visited in the afternoon and brought my laptop, wallet, some night clothes that I could easily wear to replace the hospital gown, some slippers, a few pairs of newly purchased underwear in large sizes and a wash bag from my home. I had been looking forward to receiving familiar items to introduce some normality into my day, and I was very happy to see her and chat about other things outside the hospital room. She was very pleased to hear about my progress and had arrived when I was finishing up my physio session. At least the massive underwear I had requested due to my swollen hips provided us with some comedy.

I was grateful to be still for a few hours, as I was very tired. My exercises in the hospital bed to mobilise my legs felt comparatively easier than previously, although pain levels were higher because of the physio sessions I had been doing.

The occupational therapist visited to discuss my ongoing care, the imminent arrival of my mother and a description of my home environment. There were many aspects to be considered before I could be discharged, and I was concerned they were trying to do this as quickly as possible. The flights of three stairs into my flat in addition to the steep set of narrow stairs between the mezzanine floor and open-plan living space were my main concern.

I did not see at this stage of my recovery how it would be possible to safely negotiate these. I could only just lift my toe from the floor to manage tiny steps on level ground. The sooner I could have the support of family or a close friend to be present when these decisions were being made, the better. It made me very tired having to consider the next steps, when I was still struggling just to make the first one safely each time I left the bed and stood on my feet!

15:20 Physiotherapy

This session involved a series of practical tasks. I had to try to put on my sling and a pair of slippers myself. I didn't quite manage it as I could not reach forward or bend down.

I stood up and took to the walking frame determinedly, knowing this was my last session for the day. I wanted to try to lift the toe from the floor when making my tiny 10- to 15-centimetre steps. Again, I had refused to take the liquid morphine.

My left foot responded, and after a number of steps I achieved marginal clearance over the floor on the right foot, too. The resulting spasms on the left side indicated just how much more stability was required to do this, but I was elated. It felt like another significant breakthrough, and when I had done it once, I knew I could achieve it again.

The right side was still very limited by pain through the lower back, glute and groin, but it was evident that it would respond with more practice. The pathway between brain and muscle movement in the foot had finally been painfully rewired.

My final few tasks to perform while up on my feet were firstly to sit myself in a chair beside the bed at a suitable height and then get up again independently. This was surprisingly painful due to the hip angle of 90 degrees and also sitting on the pelvic fracture site. Even on a padded chair.

The final test was for me to move into and out of the bathroom – which took some time – and use it – which took some time. So many small things I had taken for granted I now had to learn how to do again. I was pleased with my progress; finally, my brain was talking to my legs and feet again.

Friday 29 June 2012

10:30 Physiotherapy

Today's session involved being introduced to a single elbow crutch as a substitute for the walking frame. I started off by independently fitting my sling and trying to put my slippers on.

After I mustered the energy and motivation to stand up, I used the crutch in the left hand to put together more even lengthy steps as encouraged. Up until this point my left foot was taking proportionately longer steps compared to the right. I concentrated on lifting the toe each time to try and swing the leg forward and had an unsteady episode at one point.

It was a co-ordination exercise that also required balancing solely on my left leg (relatively stronger) as I transferred the right leg and crutch forward. I contemplated the ever-present pain from my back and pelvis and damage to existing injuries if I were to fall. The floor was undoubtedly hard.

I extended the walk out into the corridor and down the hall much farther than I had been before, aware of the activity and pace of doctors, other patients and visitors as I shuffled along at a snail's pace. It felt good having the freedom to walk around with the crutch rather than the cumbersome frame on wheels in front of me.

After lunch, more medication and a light rest, I had a call from my mum to let me know that she had arrived safely and was in my apartment. She would be making her way to the hospital.

15:00 Physiotherapy

A repeat of my morning walk out into the corridor with the crutch gave me the opportunity to start working on my heel-to-toe gait as I was still dragging my right foot around by the toe most of the time. Things were improving, but there was still pain and the constant fear of falling.

The physio seemed pleased with my efforts to use the single crutch instead of the walking frame. I had passed that test; the next was to climb up and down stairs.

Later that afternoon my mum finally arrived. I was so happy to see her. When my evening meal arrived, she let me know that she would bring in something more nourishing to eat the next day. Whatever it was I'd been served up wasn't something we could actually recognise.

It had been a busy day, and I was extremely tired when she left. Sleep came easily that night.

Saturday 30 June 2012

Today was a challenge of mountain-ascent proportions. Stair climb day. After the usual morning routine in the hospital ward, no doctor's rounds as it was a Saturday, it seemed fairly quiet. A wheelchair had been fetched to take me to the hospital gymnasium.

I started off with a short walk from the wheelchair to a simple stair arrangement of two steps between two parallel bars for support. My movement felt stiff as it was quite early in the morning, and I hadn't mobilised very much before the physio had arrived.

After explaining and demonstrating the process of using the crutch in combination with the right leg, stepping up off my left leg each time to ascend or descend one at a time, it was time to attempt the stair climb myself.

It was hard to believe that such a simple task could seem so difficult to achieve. Lifting the left leg up 15 centimetres to a step felt like a mammoth undertaking. I leaned heavily on the crutch for support and considered how quickly the physio's reaction times would be if I lost my balance.

I managed to co-ordinate the crutch and good (bad) leg to ascend the two stairs, pausing to stop at the top due to the wave of nausea induced by the effort and pain. For a moment or two I wasn't sure I would be able to get down and clung to the crutch, leaning against the bar.

When the room stopped spinning, I composed myself and placed the crutch on the lower step, ready to support my weight and slowly inch my injured right leg down. Bringing the left foot down to meet the right foot set off horrible movement in my lower back and pelvis accompanied by acute pain. Taking a deep breath I managed to repeat the movement and limped towards a nearby chair to sit down for a moment.

I knew I would have to master this challenge if I were to be able to manage the steps inside my flat – let alone the four flights I would have to climb to reach it in the first place.

After another two attempts to master the up and down exercise of just two stairs, with seated rests in between, I managed a short walk around the gym and then was taken back to my room in the wheelchair.

The physio suggested I might need morphine before the afternoon session.

The occupational therapist arrived soon after, and she seemed keen for me to be assessed to be discharged home after learning that my mother had arrived from Australia. There followed a lengthy discussion around the challenges of my split-level home layout and access to the apartment four flights of stairs up.

I wondered what options were available to me, apart from arranging temporary accommodation in a single-level apartment. The speed at which my return home was unfolding was worrying. I had only demonstrated a very basic level of mobility after all.

My mum arrived with lunch she had made. It was one of my favourite foods, a Thai chicken salad, with fresh herbs, vegetables and flavour. Having some real food worked its magic on my appetite while I discussed the plans being made, how the progress was being pushed along and my concerns about not being safe in key movement techniques to be discharged home to recover, unless we could find a solution to deal with the stairs.

Due to the high levels of pain I had experienced since the morning session, I declined physio treatment that afternoon, feeling an overwhelming desire to rest. I managed a short walk out and back on level ground through the corridor outside my room, with assistance from friends.

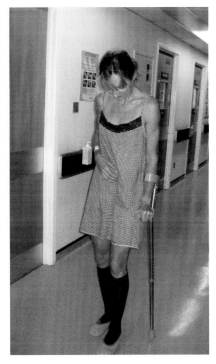

Walking progress and progression using the elbow crutch

This alleviated some of the stiffness and dull aching pain temporarily when lying still in the bed. The pain levels kept building throughout the afternoon and into the evening, and eventually I had to call for a nurse for assistance. Once given some morphine I was able to finally settle into a few hours of sleep.

It was clear I had been pushed too far, too soon, and my body really just needed to rest and regroup before pushing on to the next stage of recovery objectives so that I could go home from hospital. I couldn't believe how far I had come in a week.

In seven days my life had become unrecognisable. I was learning to walk again, managing incredible levels of pain to climb stairs. As I drifted off I wondered where I would be in another seven days.

Making the transition to the home environment:

Occupational therapist assessment aims to identify any particular requirements for home access, mobility, carrying out daily tasks and being able to live in a home environment.

Necessary equipment will usually be supplied by the hospital, arranged through local social services or the Red Cross.

Consult your GP to advise on any ongoing care, medication or further requirements for physiotherapy.

Access the College of Occupational Therapists website for further information or to locate a privately practicing OT instead of NHS OT:

www.cot.co.uk/about-ot/about-ot

Claire Cameron, *occupational therapist*

Sunday 1 July 2012

I woke feeling battered in body and foggy in mind. I recollected what had happened and made the connection it was possibly the morphine 'hangover effect'.

The morning routine of pain medications and vital sign checks proceeded then breakfast arrived. The bedwash had progressed to a shower, but it took a long time. I needed a nurse to carry or deliver my items to the shower room as I made my slow shuffle there and then to bring them back to the room afterwards.

When the physio arrived I told them the pain from stair exercise had been extreme, and I was exhausted because of poor sleep. My body needed time to regroup and repair, that much was obvious to me. I knew about pushing the body to breaking point – and I knew how to avoid it. So I opted for a day of rest. No physio exercises this morning.

After a morning resting, another homemade lunch and a visit from mum, I was wheeled off by the physio to do battle with the steps again. Triumph: I completed three reps of the stairs with only a few moments of instability and even took a few steps around the physiotherapy gym. The pain was still there, but for the most part it was masked by the morphine I was being encouraged to take.

Back in my room, after an evening meal and once my second set of visitors left, I was extremely tired and fell to asleep easily.

Monday 2 July 2012

Morning doctors' rounds update: I was expected to be discharged home in the next day or two. I still worried I would not be able to manage the stairs and raised my concerns, but it was pretty clear I was on the hospital pathway to the exit door.

12:00 – Physiotherapy

Two physios arrived for my sessions, and I was taken to a rather daunting concrete set of stairs beside the lift. Today's task: 14 steps – up and down. It would at least set me up to manage the journey into and around my apartment.

The pain set in soon after the first few steps, and I found myself counting down until I managed the two long flights – 14 steps. I looked back down with fear. It seemed a long way down, and I wasn't sure I could maintain balance and co-ordination for that distance.

With one physio ahead of me on the step below and one right behind me with arms outstretched either side of my waist, I set off slowly. The click of the crutch tapping each step, followed by my right slippered foot, then my left, made for a strange rhythm but kept me focused on the next step.

I reached the bottom of the stairs, sweating from the effort, and felt like I had climbed a mountain on my bike on one of my frequent summer training trips to the Alps. It was the breakthrough I needed. I was relived to start thinking about life back in my own home, and with support I might actually be able to function on a daily basis.

Tuesday 3 July 2012

After a lengthy morning full of admin, I was discharged from the hospital with a bag of medication, a walking crutch and a list of exercises to continue doing from the physio. I was taken by wheelchair down to the hospital entrance and sat inside the entrance, looking out at the rain while mum went and fetched my car from the car park.

When she drew up outside, I lamented I had chosen to buy a sports car, but with a considerable amount of pain I managed to lower myself into the seat. My back and pelvis were distinctly unhappy about the position they were in, but fear of climbing the stairs to my home soon overwhelmed the discomfort.

It was great to finally arrive back at my apartment. It was 10 days since the accident, and my life had completely changed.

But I wasn't there yet. Now it was time for the stairs. With a deep breath I reminded myself of the process of 'crutch first, lift right foot, left foot last'.

I carefully tackled each step on the first flight before having a short rest to get on top of the pain level.

Once up the next flight of stairs, I felt more confident, and I managed the last flight without a break so that I was standing outside the front door.

Once inside I felt as though I had been away for a long time, and everything in my familiar living environment looked a little different somehow when I returned. We set about removing hazards and trip risks, and it became clear that I would need some mobility aids to help me get around.

Finally it was time for bed, and it felt great to be back in the peace and quiet of my own home. While the bed had been fitted with a padded mattress topper to alleviate pressure on my lower back and pelvis, it wasn't quite as comfortable as the hospital air bed. However, the rewards of being home were the perfect stillness and quiet once the lights were out.

Go beyond listening to your body:

You know your body and have greater awareness of feedback from various injuries or sites than you might think. Let your body tell you where the problems are, as you go through the process of recovering and stabilising.

'Change happens when we venture over the edge and take one small step at a time.'

CHAPTER 5:
OPERATION CLAVICLE

Biggest achievement: Walking without support

Top speed: 2 kph
Elevation gain: 5 m of ascent, 3 flights of stairs
Distance: 50 m

Wednesday 4 July 2012

I felt like a stranger in my own apartment. All the things I had been able to do without so much as thinking twice about I no longer could.

The stairs were a continuous challenge. The 13 steps – an ominous number – I had to contemplate at regular intervals. My bathroom, bedroom and office were all at the top of them. I did not want to risk a fall. Memories of the acute levels of pain were still too fresh, and I didn't fancy a repeat.

The first task was to make things safe. This meant removing the dozens of pairs of trainers and cycling shoes I had left around the place. I didn't want sight of them anyway. It was a fairly brutal reminder of what I had lost, and because I didn't know if I would be doing any of those activities again, removing them from immediate view was best.

Anyway footwear with laces and clasps was a total no-go. I had only one properly working arm, and trying to push my feet into shoes just hurt my hips. In the end there were just a couple of slip on pairs that were any use to me.

Everything had to be done slowly and left-handed (I am not). I could not prepare meals for myself, eat with a knife and fork or get around very fast. It was not a speed I was used to. Efficient and quick: yes; slow: no. Occasionally I would forget my limitations and try to do something only to have the pain to stop me and hang around for ages afterwards.

Life had changed significantly, and some days it became overwhelming just how much I needed the support of family and friends to do the things I had taken for granted all my life.

In the morning my first conscious thoughts before opening my eyes were usually questions as to why I woke feeling like I had been run over by a bus during the night.

It still often took a few minutes to remember and associate the injuries I had with the accident. My body ached as soon as the pain medication wore off – at approximately four hourly intervals day and night.

I started to plan my daily activities and rehab around the pain peaks from my back, pelvis and shoulder through the day. Too much time on my feet would mean my lower back really hurt. When there was pain I had no choice but to listen to my body and try to find a way of sitting or lying to take the pressure away.

It was a matter of having to adapt quickly to learn new techniques – and that anything I wanted to be able to do would happen eventually but would generally take twice as long.

Simple things like bathing, eating at the dining room table, sitting at my desk and moving around the apartment took such effort it had to be planned.

From the first day at home I tried to reestablish some semblance of a routine, as my physical therapy was a priority. Each day involved carrying out physiotherapy exercises for 30 to 60 minutes three to five times a day, a little walking with aid of the elbow crutch around the apartment, some work and resting in the afternoons.

Fatigue levels were high and didn't take long to kick in after a spell of activity or concentration. My usually high energy levels seemed to have vanished. In short, the pain and recovering from the injuries was making me very tired.

As in hospital, my day would start with pain medication, although I was usually woken before this by the pain in my back and hips. On a few occasions, when I had to get up in the early morning, my muscles went into spasms, and I was unable to move. I found myself stuck, balanced on a crutch and trying to manage the pain. I resorted to the breathing techniques Debbie had taught me at the scene of the accident.

It took 20 to 30 minutes for me to activate my leg muscles in bed to initiate the challenge and process of getting up in the morning.

I used a range of bed-bound exercise progressions that had been my physiotherapy while in hospital. They all involved simple movements, engaging the feet, ankles, hamstrings, quadriceps, gluteal muscles and hip flexors.

Just getting out of bed and then standing up always felt like a huge achievement. Once I started slowly moving off towards the door I would notice how gradually I could lengthen my steps from 3 to 5 centimetres to 10 to 15 centimetres as my muscles let go of some of the tension stored in them. I figured it was the extent of the repair work going on overnight while I slept that meant my legs, back and hips felt as though they had 'shut down' in the mornings.

Getting dressed was the next challenge. Identifying suitable garments to wear with shoulder, back and leg restrictions narrowed my choice on any given day. It took up to two hours to get myself ready and make the careful descent stiffly downstairs for breakfast.

Morning after clavicle operation

Saturday 7 July 2012

The first weekend back in my own home came and went.

Having my routine changed completely took some adjustment. I tried not to think about events I had entered for on Sunday and the following weekends throughout the summer. The prospect provoked too many questions about whether I would ever have the opportunity to train and compete again. It also led to inevitable comparisons of how I was spending my time and what I would have been doing if I were preparing for a race.

For the first time I didn't mind being indoors most of the time. I was anxious and worried about going out because I felt defenceless. This was a new experience for me. It was good to have chats on Skype and visits from friends to look forward to.

One of the best things about being home was saying goodbye to the hospital food. I could eat things I recognised again. Every day my mum presented one of my favourite breakfasts: fresh fruit, berries, nuts, seeds and natural yoghurt or eggs, mushrooms and tomatoes.

Over breakfast and the morning news mum would plan the other meals that day and ingredients we might need to source. Fortunately my mother is a very talented cook and always uses fresh ingredients.

The food she prepared contained high levels of antioxidants and nutrients essential to helping the body recover. Meals included high-quality sources of protein to rebuild or help to offset the significant muscle loss and atrophy from the reduced activity. Salads and main meals were made up of more than 10 vegetables, enhanced with fresh herbs.

My fundamental belief as an athlete of quality sources of fuel being required for the best training and racing had now become even more important. I saw food as my medicine. The sound nutrition required to support my recovery from the inside out was the same as a menu of unrefined, fresh food providing energy and nutrients to support a high training load to recover well for the next session.

Benefits of eating unprocessed and 'real' food:

Choosing to eat unprocessed and unrefined food requires more planning and preparation; however, it is well worth the effort required.

Opting for grain-free provides more space on your plate for nutrient-rich vegetables, fruit and protein sources and for essential amino acids such as meat or fish.

Benefits – for an athlete:

Consistency in energy levels throughout the day – less likely to suffer afternoon 'lag' in energy

Sustained high quality of training sessions, particularly relevant in peak training volume phases requiring multiple sessions per day

Facilitating or improving immune system health, being less likely to succumb to illnesses or infections, allowing continuity in training and therefore enhanced progression

Prevention of injuries and increased rate of recovery from high-intensity and endurance sessions due to the full profile of amino acids and complete proteins gained from eating a range of meat, fish, chicken and eggs

Benefits – for recovery from serious injuries:

Positive impact on appetite to encourage regular eating patterns, increased appeal to senses of freshly prepared foods, in taste, aroma and textures (Opiate pain medication can suppress the appetite.)

Improved feeling of energy during late mornings and afternoons, when fatigue levels are high as pain levels increase and medication starts to wear off

Boosting mitochondria and ability of cells to regenerate and heal injuries, due to substantial levels of antioxidant intake from real food

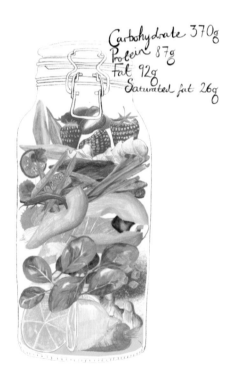

Carbohydrate 370g
Protein 87g
Fat 92g
Saturated fat 26g

Choosing to eat locally sourced, unprocessed, seasonal food yields greater nutrient content than processed, convenient options for eating.

Tips to optimise nutrition during recovery:

Planning – Create a healthy daily or weekly menu, listing ingredients. Eliminate processed foods from your cupboards, fridge and pantry.

Preparation – Cook healthy meals from fresh ingredients and freeze additional quantities. If unable to prepare yourself in the short term, create a schedule or rota of willing friends and family to bring in freshly prepared meals for you.

Produce – Fresh is best. Try home delivery from farm or organic produce suppliers. Aim to use mostly local produce when possible. Online supermarket home delivery services are helpful, too. Source seasonal produce to ensure it has the highest possible nutrient value. Avoid foods that have been transported long distances, kept in storage or artificially ripened with chemicals.

Table 1

RECOVERY MEAL PLANNER			
Wake-up	Breakfast	Lunch	Dinner
Juice – Orange: orange, ginger, turmeric, carrot	Quinoa and linseed porridge with berries and hazelnuts	Mushroom and spring onion omelette and roasted tomato salad	Roasted lemon and thyme chicken with vegetables
Juice – Beet: beetroot, apple, parsley, lime or lemon	Scrambled eggs, with mushrooms and tomatoes	Chicken and celeriac soup	Baked salmon sesame with salad
Juice – Berry: strawberries or raspberries, mint, cucumber, acacia	Spinach, basil, spring onion and egg-baked pots	Salmon, avocado, celeriac sushi	Thai beef salad
Juice – Green: kale or spinach, apple, grapes, celery, ginger	Bircher muesli seeds, flaked almonds, grated apple, coconut or greek yoghurt, berries	Roasted butternut squash, tomato, avocado and tuna salad	Mediterranean chicken, pesto and vegetables
Juice – Citrus: lemon, lime, orange, celery, pear	Eggplant (aubergine) toast topped with spinach, prosciutto and boiled eggs	Halloumi, sweet potato, sprout, almond and pear salad	Haddock gratin: spinach, haddock, mashed celeriac and parsnip

Monday 9 July 2012

11:20 Hospital outpatient appointment

After my first week at home, I had a return visit to the hospital as an outpatient to check on the healing progress of the pelvis and clavicle fractures. However, when I arrived I discovered only my pelvis was to be checked.

The consultant expected I would need to wait a few more weeks or perhaps months for the collarbone to begin to mend and become more stable. This was news to me.

As I discussed the pelvic X-rays it became obvious the delay in reviewing my shoulder was because I couldn't move due to my pelvis and sacrum injuries. I tried to point out that even getting back a small amount of movement would allow me to resume some of my work.

Waiting as much as six months for a shattered clavicle to mend itself when the broken bone ends were fractured and separated by 2 centimetres and overlapping by 1 centimetre (as shown on the X-ray images) was not a realistic option for an athlete who wanted to have a functional shoulder once healed. I was concerned about how much the clavicle would be shortened as I viewed the June and July X-rays side by side. Suboptimal shoulder function and implications for shoulder, back and posture were obvious. Eight weeks of recovery time, a clavicle with non-union: it was time for a second medical opinion.

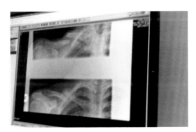

Clavicle X-rays showing initial fracture and resultant non-union overlap at 6 weeks

Tuesday 10 July 2012

First week after leaving hospital progress report: walking with crutch 20 metres a minute on level surface, slow but steady.

What was soon becoming a standard day for me started with 20 to 30 minutes of my exercises in bed. The range of motion was starting to improve, and I was now pushing through the pain barrier before the medication started to work.

Breakfast and planning the day usually revolved around any medical appointments, the daily menu and visitors.

I would manage to complete an hour or two at my desk before discomfort overcame productivity. A post-lunch rest had become essential to deal with the rising fatigue levels by then.

The amount of rest depended on levels of activity. Afternoon exercises and a short walk outside – with the three-flight stair climb up and down – meant more rest was needed. Dinner and an early night would be a welcome finish to the day.

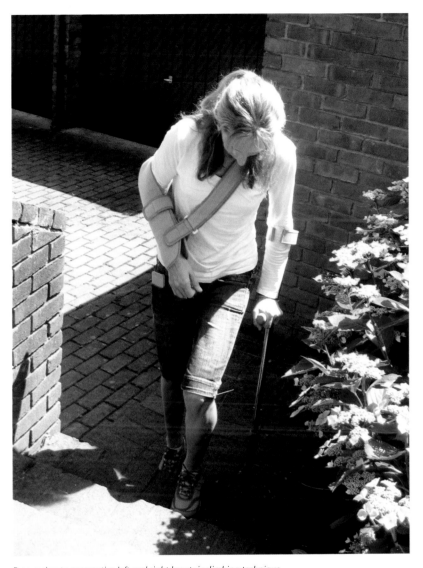

Progressing to consecutive left and right leg stair climbing technique

Wednesday 11 July 2012

20:30 Physiotherapy appointment

There was noticeable improvement. As I arrived for the appointment and got myself out of the car and shuffled the 30 metres across the car park I could see the progress I was making. It was hard to believe the accident was less than three weeks ago, and I was more or less able to walk.

I worked with the same physiotherapist as in hospital, and she encouraged me to build upon the exercises I was completing at least three times a day.

Armed with some new movement patterns to address some of the everyday challenges of compromised function, I shuffled back to the carpark and the waiting car with my mum at the wheel.

Thursday 12 July 2012

My mother left on her long flight back to Sydney. I was on my own. It was a daunting prospect, even though she had helped fill the freezer with prepared meals and plan weekly grocery shopping deliveries.

My father was planning to arrive in 10 days. It was a long time when only one of your limbs works properly. This would be a huge challenge.

I still hadn't adjusted to my damaged body limitations. My legs were slowly learning to walk again; I was restricted by one arm in a sling and unable to lift, carry or bend. It meant I would have to ask for help. This was not my strong suit.

That afternoon a good friend brought my bikes back. They had been taken away and stored overnight by a local cyclist on the day of the accident.

It was very strange to watch them being unloaded from his car and wheeled to my garage. I didn't feel comfortable at all, seeing my race bike for the first time since the accident.

I couldn't assemble either of the bikes, which had been packed down to travel, or even wheel them into the garage.

However, I did check my race bike thoroughly. It was also a casualty of the accident. The sight of the buckled rear wheel, long slide mark on the tyre and scratched frame where it had met the road on its right side made me feel sick and sweaty.

Unexpectedly I found myself replaying the accident in my head. While the bike was damaged it had fared better than I had. I had effectively cushioned the blow.

A wave of exhaustion hit me hard that evening, fuelled by deep-seated injury pain from an active day. I had lost my appetite again and tried to eat an evening meal, but it was a matter of routine rather than hunger.

Accident flashbacks kept waking me during the night. I relived the events leading up to the smash, tried to reason why and at one point woke thinking I was still in the hospital. By the time morning came I felt I had not slept at all.

Table 2

DAY IN THE LIFE OF RECOVERY	
Day in the life of injured athlete	Day in the life of athlete
Saturday 14 July 2012	*Saturday 9 July 2011*
6:00 – Early morning bed exercises	6:00 – Wake and leave for training
7:00 – Breakfast and medication	6:25 – Masters swim session
8:15 – Taxi arrives	8:00 – Shower, change
8:30 – Hydrotherapy session with physiotherapist	8:15 – Breakfast
9:00 – Taxi home	9:30 – Endurance bike-and-run combination session (6 hours)
10:00 – Coffee and catch-up with friend preparing lunch in advance	90-mile cycle into 4-5 mile run
11:00 – Skype parents in Australia, update on progress since mum left on Thursday	15:30 – Arrive home, recovery snack, shower and change
12:00 – Medication and physio exercises	17:00 – Stretch and recovery time
	18:30 – Evening meal
13:00 – Lunch	21:00 – Bed
14:00 – Rest	Key training day – 2 weeks before winning middle distance event
15:00-16:00 – Medication and physio exercises	Fambridge Yacht Haven Triathlon in 4:31
17:00 – Friend arrives; accompanied evening walk outside, 30 min	
18:00 – Help to prepare evening meal; dinner	
20:00 – Physio exercises and medication	
20:30 – Prepare for bed by 21:00-21:30	
Key success today – first hydrotherapy session	

Sunday 15 July 2012

I woke to the reality of not racing on a Sunday morning but philosophically applied myself to my morning exercises. It was getting easier to move, but I still had to tackle pain, spasms and the difficulty of moving heavy, injured limbs.

My morning ritual of limbering up the muscles and gentle movement took 30 to 45 minutes each day. I looked forward to seeing the progress made each time as I worked through painful movement to a more manageable level of operating limbs and body.

Morning activation ritual:

1. Lying down – stretching legs from hips; pointing toes, isolating one leg at a time and moving side to side as far as pain allows

2. Lying down – bending knees and straightening each leg in isolation

3. Lying down – lifting and lowering straight legs with toes pulled towards the shin and foot straight

4. Lying down – knees bent, feet at hip width; activating glutes and core muscles to flatten lower back into the floor or bed

5. Lying down – legs straight and stretched; push knees into bed to activate thighs and glutes

6. Sitting – lifting and straightening one leg at a time

7. Sitting – lifting one leg at a time in hip flexion, knee bent

8. Standing – one-leg side lifts; holding on to support for balance

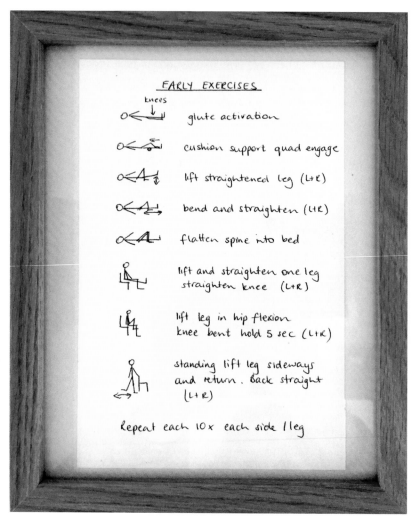

Key exercises as prescribed by physiotherapist, framed and hung on a wall as a constant reminder to repeat each day

The routine of friends coming in the mornings and afternoons to help was working well. It helped to structure the day around my own physiotherapy exercise routine three or four times a day and the evening walk. A rota ensured I had a regular visit by friends in the morning and afternoons. Many of them offered to cook and bring in prepared evening meals or unpack shopping if I had scheduled a delivery and needed a hand. Lifting, carrying or bending down were all significant challenges with multiple fractures.

While I could now walk without a crutch inside my home for around 20 metres (grabbing furniture along the way), I didn't feel confident leaving the apartment on my own.

This was mainly due to the flights of stairs outside which still presented painful challenges. Careful co-ordination of a crutch, functional leg and non-functional leg was required.

Having one arm in a sling meant saving myself in the event of a fall would be extremely difficult. I was, however, getting more used to little mishaps and dealing with them without overreacting and subsequent painful consequences.

Monday 16 July 2012

A morning outpatient appointment for new X-rays showed the fracture of the pelvis and sacrum was slowly healing. I hoped this would provide more stability as time went on, and the consultant seemed very confident that it would mend well.

My concern was over the lack of symmetry and implications for sport. However, this was quickly dismissed. He was also not willing to X-ray the clavicle despite my obvious and ongoing concerns.

For a week I settled into my new routines with visits from friends and my focus on increasing my physio exercises to four or five times each day.

My aim was to keep making progress between my two, weekly physio appointments. I extended the recommended exercises provided by my therapist with my own research and reading of articles about similar injuries. I put together a hydrotherapy session based on most of my land-based exercises to try in the water.

My local pool offered hydrotherapy sessions much like a swimming timetable with public opening times for a limited period each day. I arranged a taxi to collect me to and from these sessions and put together a series of weekly sessions to work through.

Almost immediately I noticed the significant benefits of improved mobility, progressing my walking technique and range and best of all, reduced pain levels afterwards for many hours.

The Tour de France was providing a good incentive for me to rest in the afternoons on the sofa, watching the cyclists tackle mountains in the Alps I had ridden many times. A few of my triathlon and cycling friends timed their afternoon visits to watch stages with me.

It had been one month of living with my injuries and recovering to a point where I looked forward to my physical therapy every day and to seeing the improvements made. I was seeing the hospital physiotherapist twice a week and was also doing hydrotherapy. Doing simple exercises supported by the heated water brought incredible pain relief. It also gave me a familiar routine and replaced my five swim training sessions a week.

I had taken to going for an evening walk; it was just a lap of the garden. This evening's took 30 minutes, and I managed consistent heel to toe walking with similar length strides on both left and right for 50 metres. I took two rests.

Hydrotherapy benefits:

It improves recovery by facilitating movement range while injured supported by the water.

The warm water temperature (34°C) promotes circulation around the body, speeding up repair to injury sites.

Water pressure keeps swelling around the injuries to a minimum.

Sports-specific movement patterns can be reintroduced in the water to build strength and function at low intensity and without impact.

A minimum of 20 to 30 minutes three times per week every other day reduces or helps manage high pain levels.

The properties of water allow controlled loading of muscles and ligaments, allowing functional patterns of load to be practiced and developed.

30-minute hydrotherapy session:

Aims: engaging and moving legs in small movements using hips and core

Hydrotherapy session:
Warm-up for 5 minutes

Walking up and down the pool forwards and backwards and then side to side

Moving slowly forwards and backwards in hip to chest deep water for 5 to 10 minutes

Approximately 10 metres in distance, moving at a rate that is slightly challenging to engage legs forward with water resistance

Standing with hands on a float and arms straight and moving the float from centre of body to left, side, back to centre and then to right

Stretching and strengthening exercises for 15 to 20 minutes:

Facing the wall holding on to the side of pool or support bars at chest or hip height swing one leg forwards, backwards and sideways.

Facing away from the wall and using the bars or long noodle float for balance, lift hips and cycle legs in the water.

Using a float in front of the body, kick from the hips with legs straight to move forwards through the pool.

Cool-down, 5 minutes

Walking up and down the pool forwards and backwards, side to side as per warm-up

Benefits:

Improved circulation and reduced pain post session

Ease of access – automatic doors in and out

Much easier, safer and more spacious showering and changing areas compared with home environment

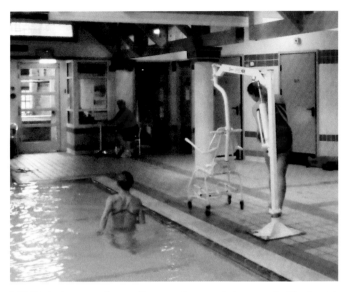

Initial hydrotherapy sessions working on water-supported movement without crutch

Sunday 22 July 2012

I decided to return to one of my favourite work activities and run one of my weekend swim workshops with the help of my assistant coach.

We worked out how much help I would need, including being driven to and from the venue, setting up and carrying equipment, filming swimmers under water and walking up and down the poolside.

I delivered the session but was left utterly exhausted and experienced high levels of back, shoulder and hip pain for days afterwards. Weight-bearing for long periods of time hurt.

I learned an important lesson that day and that was to make connections between my rate of pain and improvement to training principles I had used over the years.

Just as in conditioning progression for sport, gradual increases needed to be carefully planned for me to make the transition back into my normal active life.

Whether it was a slight overreach or major undertaking, as my first day back on the pool deck at work showed, I would suffer significant setbacks afterwards as my injuries and body would be less able to manage simple tasks.

I would have to factor in a few easier days to be able to pick up the rehab process back where I had been.

Thankfully my father arrived from Australia later that day, and I was was very relieved to have his help.

My coaching work creating training plans was limited to a few hours at my desk when the pain medication worked effectively during the day. With assistance, I adapted and rearranged my home office environment to allow me to sit at my desk for longer periods of time. Sitting and trying to type with my sling on was painful, and there was no easy way to support the arm. My shoulders and back would ache from the effort.

Sunday 29 July 2012

The anniversary of last year's win at a middle-distance race was spent in the usual routine of mobility exercises, medication, eating, resting and more mobility exercises.

I tried to avoid thinking about races I wasn't on the start line for on my now abandoned plan for the season.

The London 2012 Olympics and cycle road race was passing just by my house, and it presented incentive to leave the house. I was driven in my car a short 400 metres to the end of the road where the riders would whizz past. I would find it too far to walk each way and spend half an hour or more standing up on my feet to watch the race.

Standing among the crowds was quite terrifying. I was unable to move quickly and feared getting knocked and losing my balance in the excitement of the race passing. After watching the peloton fly past, travelling the very route I took the day of the accident, I was very grateful to be transported the 400 metres home in the car again.

Wednesday 1 August 2012

A few days later when the Olympic time trial passed right by my home, I had a better opportunity to enjoy all the action. A group of friends came over for lunch and gathered chairs, effectively securing an area right outside my front gate. It was safe and very easy for me to retreat indoors. It was a much better experience although it still left me incredibly tired afterwards. I started to wonder if it was the pain medication that constantly made me feel like sleeping. A correlation between taking the medication and needing to sleep was becoming clear.

Friday 3 August 2012

A few weeks after my first attempt to return to coaching, I planned to take one of the evening swim squad sessions despite the high risk of falling on the wet, slippery pool deck. I decided that I would try to deliver the session in a limited capacity, seated in a chair if necessary.

Although everything took a long time with one arm and a crutch, it felt a great achievement to be back on the pool deck. Seeing my athletes, the progress made in the few weeks I had been away and immersing myself in the familiar routine and process of delivering a session provided a healthy distraction from the reality, difficulty and pain of my situation.

Although exhausted afterwards, I resolved to try to coach at least one evening squad session each week. A coaching session triggered high pain levels for 24 hours afterwards, and I would need to plan in quieter days afterwards.

It was overwhelming, after anything I did, just how much support was offered before, during and after these sessions from my close group of friends and athletes.

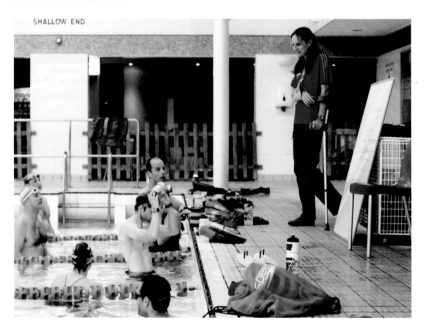

Squad coaching with mobility support plan in place

Monday 6 August 2012

My birthday was spent having a six-week follow-up appointment at the hospital as an outpatient. The X-rays showed the clavicle had not healed at all, but the pelvic fractures were starting to mend. I asked for my records be transferred to a local hospital.

The first important element to address was my appointment with the consultant shoulder surgeon for a second opinion on how likely the clavicle was to mend on its own.

Six weeks had elapsed since the accident, and the shoulder felt like it was frozen to protect the separated bones. The consultant made a quick assessment of the X-ray and said surgery would be required to plate the clavicle together so it could mend.

I was booked in for surgery on the following morning at 7 am.

Tuesday, 7 August 2012

After a very early start at 4 am, we arrived at the hospital at 7 am by taxi. The pre-operation preparation went calmly although I got a little emotional bidding my father farewell and shuffling off to the waiting room.

I climbed onto a trolley and was soon hooked up to a number of sensors and monitors. A large arrow, pointing to the correct shoulder, was drawn on my right arm. It was probably best they didn't get the wrong one. I only had one functioning arm after all.

The pre-anaesthetic soon had me drifting off mid conversation. I woke in recovery, aware of a strangely heavy shoulder.

After a while one of the nurses checked on me and explained I would be soon transferred to a room. I was very surprised to see it was 17:30 – most of the day had disappeared whilst I was under the knife.

The surgery was successful, and my clavicle had been successfully put back together. I was left to rest and sleep and looked forward to going home the next morning.

At 5 am I was woken by unbearable pain, which would not go despite medication. By 7 am it was intolerable, and I was given some morphine to try to bring the threshold back to a manageable level. From this point I was advised to take the medication regularly for the next two to three days.

I was reminded of the consultant's words before surgery. He said he would mend my clavicle, but he would not be my friend afterwards because of the pain it would cause. How right he was.

By mid-morning my father arrived, and preparations were made to take me home by taxi. It had taken a long time to wash and get dressed, even with a nurse helping. I had made the mistake of lifting my right arm slightly and ended up doubled over in pain with gritted teeth until it subsided sufficiently to ring the buzzer for help.

I was dispatched with a supply of morphine and my 'regular' daily doses of tramadol, paracetamol and ibuprofen to keep me going for a week. A follow-up appointment as an outpatient would be required in the coming weeks to monitor how effectively the plate was managing to help the fracture heal. A physio popped in to advise on restrictions in range of motion to shoulder level, including not carrying anything for at least six weeks.

The one-hour taxi ride home was dire. I was in a lot of pain, and typically a London taxi driver wanted to take as many back streets as possible (speed humps, agony).

I went straight to bed when I arrived back at the apartment and spent the next 24 hours dozing then waking in pain.

I needed the prescribed morphine early in the morning once again to gain some respite and then stay on top of the threshold of intolerable pain.

I emerged from the experience of surgery with a much more stable shoulder, manageable pain levels, and with what I hoped was the worst of the physical recovery behind me. The three-day post-surgery nightmare soon became a painful blur in my memory.

Post-surgery tips:

Expect high fatigue levels afterwards; it is the body's response to the stress of the surgery.

The systemic inflammatory response causes the fatigue and sometimes flu-like feelings during recovery; all of your energy stores are being mobilised to start healing.

Allow for adaptation and the body repairing itself.

Appreciate your body has switched from an anabolic to catabolic state, and your inflammatory mediators, stress hormones, adrenaline and immune modulators are in temporary overdrive.

Try to be up and mobile as soon as possible to help restore normal bodily functions.

Seek advice from your GP or the consultant or surgeon if you have complications after surgery.

Kate McCombe, *consultant anaesthetist, Frimley Park Hospital*

> *'Seek the very best quality nutrition for recovery to promote healing from the inside out.'*

CHAPTER 6:
FUNCTIONAL MOVEMENT

Biggest achievement: Covering more than a few metres at a time by mobility scooter

Top speed: 3 kph
Elevation gain: 5 m, up stairs to apartment
Distance: 14 km

Friday 23 August 2012

Painful though it was, surgery resulted in much greater shoulder and spine stability once the bone and plate knitted together.

I managed to follow the physiotherapist's advice to limit arm movement below the shoulder until the broken clavicle bonded. It was pretty easy when using the arm and shoulder in any way was very painful.

After only four weeks the arm felt a lot better than it had before surgery.

The thick metal plate that had been inserted was long and protruded, making the collarbone appear very close to the skin's surface. However, its supportive role moved the recovery process forward immensely.

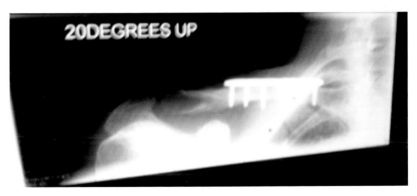

One successfully repaired right clavicle

After two weeks on 'no getting the wound wet' orders, I was delighted to get back to hydrotherapy sessions and start working on upper-body and back in addition to my hip and leg rehab exercises.

After eight weeks I could gently lift my arm above my shoulder. It was a significant point in my recovery. While it was all still very sore, at last I could put on shoes, eat with a knife and fork and wash and dry my hair in a shower. Huge steps forward in everyday life.

My father went back to Australia at the end of August, and I focused on being able to look after myself. I had an outing or two to develop confidence outside the house.

A visit to Hampton Court Palace for a few hours left me needing a three-hour rest in the afternoon. A trip to Kew Gardens was easier. Mobility scooters on offer there meant I could be out and about for longer. It was great to be outside connecting with the natural environment. The little outings were great leaps forward in terms of recovery.

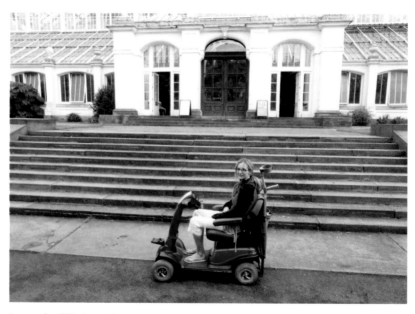

Increased mobility by scooter

Gradually my independence and confidence returned. I was under pressure to try and rebuild some of my business activities and coaching as fatigue, pain levels and time taken out of the week to attend multiple medical appointments permitted. This was a constant driving force behind everything I did to keep moving forward. It was a full-time focus finding ways to get back to what I knew, loved and wanted from life.

Short-term support post surgery:

1. Draw up a weekly rota of friends and family to assist with preparation of daily meals.

2. Arrange grocery deliveries each week; choose a company who will deliver to your kitchen (if you cannot carry heavy items for a few weeks), not just to your front door.

3. Treat yourself to a hairdresser appointment for a weekly shampoo (and blow dry) following the 'keep surgery wound dry' advice after surgery.

4. Set a non-negotiable routine; your physiotherapy exercises are your new 'training' sessions.

5. Stay positive and focus on small, incremental gains you make week on week.

6. Track progress (e.g., less pain, increased range of movement, new mastery of skills or co-ordination).

7. Use taxi services for hospital outpatient appointments and physiotherapy sessions.

Thursday 27 September 2012 – 3 months after accident

My physiotherapy sessions were progressing the range of functional movement within each injury site, with separate appointments for each injury being looked at in isolation by a range of very helpful physiotherapists. After arranging a referral through my GP, I received a short course of hydrotherapy sessions with a physiotherapist and then continued to attend two to three sessions each week.

There was a direct correlation between the time I spent working on supported movement in water and reduced pain and circulation resulting in the hours after my sessions. I started to plan my hydrotherapy sessions on or directly following days I worked more hours or were likely to have pain implications from increasing the amount of time on my feet. This approach worked effectively as my local pool had a public session in the hydrotherapy pool available most days for a few hours.

After a six-week wait, I also managed to gain a referral to work with a hydrotherapy specialist who assessed my needs, worked with me for a limited number of sessions and designed a program to continue with. After a few guided sessions I had new challenges to work with, controlling limbs in the water unsupported by the wall or floor to perform subtle movements using the core, back and hip muscles. The warmth of the water and working through greater range of movement and mobilisation always provided pain relief afterwards. I greatly looked forward to my hydro and water-based sessions; they were regular highlights each and every week.

Between my own designed hydrotherapy research and specialist input with specific exercises designed to rehabilitate each specific injury site, I had a comprehensive programme I could implement in a regular pool as well.

Gradually I resumed more of my coaching work as the Autumn months set in. My routine and workload had changed to incorporate more rest between physical time on my feet, and I would often require one to two hours of sleep in the afternoons to recover for an evening coaching session. I maintained my independent physical therapy sessions three to four times each day at home as 30- to 45-minute movement sessions based on a range of physio exercises.

Progress in movement range was slow but translated to mobility and speed to join multiple complex movements together. Everyday challenges like the stairs started to become easier. I learned to 'heel to toe' walk on my right leg, utilising the foot, ankle and hips correctly with great concentration at first. First thing in the morning these movements were always painful and required more focus to execute effective movement in a sequence. It felt very strange to have to think in order to walk correctly!

I worked hard on developing the same evenness in my gait that I had taken for granted running at three-hour marathon pace or walking for leisure. It took many weeks traipsing up and down a flat 20-metre stretch of lawn in my garden to achieve a walking gait without my walking stick or crutch. I aimed to match my right leg stride length with the consistent, even steps set by my left leg.

It felt a great achievement to have the confidence to walk outside without my trusty crutch, three months on. It provided a secure aid for mobility, particularly on stairs I still felt vulnerable without it. As my co-ordination and ability to lift the right leg improved I started to challenge myself to walk up the stairs consecutively, rather than one step at a time. It was amazing how much concentration was required to ensure my right leg and hip lifted when I needed it to engage, requiring constantly pushing through pain levels that were just about manageable. Every movement involved pain and discomfort, particularly from my lower back, right hip and leg. I was acutely aware at times that the significant level of pain medication I was taking morning, noon, afternoon and evening was helping me immeasurably improve mobility and facilitating a return to independently living most of the time.

If I did too much time on feet or overstretch my movement range, the injury sites would flare up with acute pain when lying or sitting or become aggravated as I moved. This impacted simple things like bending down to pick up an item or putting on my own shoes and socks. Sitting for long periods of time or in extreme hip flexion greater than 90 degrees proved uncomfortable.

The impact on every aspect of my life was significant; continually learning to adapt and change was key to being able to regularly identify the positive aspects under the circumstances. It could always be worse, and I often thought back to the moments lying on the road fearful that I would never again be independent or active in daily life. This kept me going, a goal on the horizon that I would eventually get back to leading an active life.

Strategies for coping:

Recognise negative thoughts that could lead towards a downward spiral.

Address negativity by focusing on what you can do, instead of issues, pain and barriers.

Maintain good health during the recovery process; look after yourself.

Eat healthily for energy and repair, not comfort.

Adhere to all medical instructions; complete physiotherapy at least as prescribed.

Have a regular sleep pattern.

Set up a weekly routine with a balance of rehabilitation, appointments, social time and admin tasks.

Seek expert advice to ease anxiety about the healing process and whether it is on track.

A lot of athlete post-injury anxiety stems from fear of reinjury; don't feel pressured to do more than you feel you are ready to physically undertake based on other people's expectations or needs.

Progress was a non-linear process that was unpredictable most days and best considered over a longer term to appreciate. My training diary was adapted to record my rehabilitation and progress, measured in metrics of mobility success rather than distance, wattage, HR intensities or time on legs.

Monday	Tuesday	Wednesday	Thursday	Friday	Saturday	Sunday	Week Summary		
Jul 25	**26**	**27**	**28**	**29**	**30**	**31**	**Jul 25 - Jul 31**		
Day off rest day	Swim P: 1:30:00 P: 4000 m Warm up 400 FC 8x50 kick w/ fins 4x100 IM 2x200 pull ... More >>	Strength P: 45.0 min Lat PD Leg press Cable adductor/ abductor Overhead pull down sing... More >>	Swim P: 1:00:00 P: 3000 m Feltham session 8:30 to 10pm OR own session: Warm up 400 ... More >>	Bike WU 15 mins Into 5x5 min Z3-4 HR efforts @ 260-280W 1 min spin rec ... More >>	Run P: 2:45:00 Double run day Run 1 (am) 1 hour 40 mins at brisk endurance pac... More >>	Run P: 30.0 min 30 mins off the bike 2.5 laps of lake passy ~2.5k loops 2 x laps a... More >>		Planned	Completed
							Total time	18:20:00	13:27:16
							Swim Dur	6:00:00	1:00:00
							Bike Dur	7:20:00	7:22:16
							Run Dur	4:15:00	4:05:00
							Strength ...	0:45:00	1:00:00
							Swim Dis	13100 m	2400 m
						C: 0:30:00	Weekly Goals		More >>
Aug 01	**02**	**03**	**04**	**05**	**06**	**07**	**Aug 01 - Aug 07**		
Run P: 1:10:00 Warm up 20 minutes, build pace easily Main set: 5 x 1600m @ tempo... C: 1:10:00 Post: 5 reps - More >>	Run P: 40.0 min 40-45 mins off the bike Bike P: 3:00:00 P: 80.00 km 3 hour ride at steady endurance More >>	Run P: 1:00:00 warm up 15- 20 mins Into 8 x 3 min hill climb reps, 3 min easy rec ... C: 1:45:00 More >>	Day off rest day Other Yoga session 6:30-8pm C: 1:15:00 Post: Steph yoga session at pure fit gym More >>	Swim P: 1:00:00 wetsuit practice Bike P: 5:30:00 5 to 5.5 hour endurance ride 2 cols tbc More >>	Bike P: 2:00:00 WU/ CD 20- 30 mins Into 6 x 8 min tempo efforts / L3W with 5 min re... C: 1:20:00 Post: 4x6-8 More >>	Run P: 2:15:00 2 - 2h 15min at marathon pace At 30, 60, 90 minutes incorporate 3 C: 2:20:00 Post: Altitude More >>		Planned	Completed
							Total time	22:50:00	22:15:33
							Swim Dur	4:30:00	4:10:00
							Bike Dur	11:15:00	10:57:33
							Run Dur	5:35:00	5:53:00
							Strength ...	1:30:00	
							Other Dur		1:15:00
							Swim Dis	6800 m	11400 m
							Weekly Goals		More >>
08	**09**	**10**	**11**	**12**	**13**	**14**	**Aug 08 - Aug 14**		
Bike P: 2:00:00 2 hour tempo ride to Passy and back w/ Rob C: 2:00:00 Swim P: 45.0 min Recovery More >>	Day off Travel to Heathrow - flight at 12pm Stretching session 30-45 mins	Run P: 1:00:00 P: 12.00 km Warm up 15 mins, into 3 x 7.5 mins at tempo pace, 2.5 min jog rec ... C: 1:00:00 More >>	Brick P: 1:10:00 WU 15 mins Into 4 x 5 min tempo efforts, at 230-250w, 2 min spin r... C: 0:55:00 C: 31.00 km	Run P: 45.0 min 45 min easy paced run C: 0:50:00 Post: feeling tired! Swim P: 1:00:00 own session	Bike P: 2:00:00 90 mins to 2 hour endurance ride C: 1:45:00 Post: felt quite tired - easy paced More >>	Run P: 1:00:00 WU 10-15 mins Into 30-45 mins @ tempo pace CD 15 mins C: 1:10:00 Post: Easy run over to More >>		Planned	Completed
							Total time	14:35:00	14:10:00
							Swim Dur	4:25:00	3:10:00
							Bike Dur	4:00:00	4:20:00
							Run Dur	2:45:00	3:30:00
							Brick Dur	1:10:00	0:55:00
							Strength ...	0:45:00	0:45:00
							Other Dur	1:30:00	1:30:00
							Weekly Goals		More >>
15	**16**	**17**	**18**	**19**	**20**	**21**	**Aug 15 - Aug 21**		
Other Taper week #2 RACE WEEK Re-check all your race needs and requireme... Strength P: 45.0 min More >>	Bike P: 45.0 min Short 45 min spin, check race bike Predominantl y L3w include 3-5 x... C: 0:45:00	Swim P: 1:00:00 P: 3000 m Warm up 400 FC 4x50m as kick/ drill into FC, off 10 sec rest 200m ... C: 1:00:00 More >>	Day off travel to Vichy Other weds- saturday Run Easy run to stretch out the legs More >>	Brick P: 30.0 min 15-20 minute spin, first thing in the morning Check wheels, bike e... C: 0:45:00 Post: 30 min More >>	Day off Aim to be off your feet for as much of the day as possible, keep l... Other weds- saturday	Race 2.6m Swim, 112m Bike, 26.2m Run C: 10:42:00 Post: 4th female and pro ~ times / splits were: Swim 1:09		Planned	Completed
							Total time	3:50:00	15:22:00
							Swim Dur	1:20:00	1:30:00
							Bike Dur	0:45:00	0:45:00
							Run Dur	0:30:00	1:00:00
							Brick Dur	0:30:00	0:45:00
							Race Dur		10:42:00
							Strength ...	0:45:00	0:40:00
							Weekly Goals		More >>

Training log comparison July 2011 with July 2012

118

Monday	Tuesday	Wednesday	Thursday	Friday	Saturday	Sunday	Week Summary		
Jul 30	31	Aug 01	02	03	04	05	Jul 30 - Aug 05		
Custom Physio exercises 3-4 x per day (30 mins) + evening walk C: 1:30:00	Other Hydro session Teddington pool C: 0:30:00 Custom Physio exercises 3-4 More >>	Custom Physio exercises 3-4 x per day (30 mins) + evening walk C: 1:30:00	Other Hydro session Teddington pool C: 0:30:00 Custom Physio exercises 3-4 More >>	Custom Physio exercises 3-4 x per day (30 mins) + evening walk C: 1:30:00	Other Hydro session Teddington pool C: 0:30:00 Custom Physio exercises 3-4 More >>	Custom Physio exercises 3-4 x per day (30 mins) + evening walk C: 1:30:00		Completed	
							Total time	12:00:00	
							Custom Dur	10:30:00	
							Other Dur	1:30:00	
							Weekly Goals	More >>	
06	07	08	09	10	11	12	Aug 06 - Aug 12		
Other Guildford hosp Fracture clinic Xrays Custom Physio exercises 3-4 x per day (30 mins) + afternoon More >>	Other UCLH hiosp app - DR Cobiella 2nd opinion on clavicle fracture Custom Physio exercises 3-4 More >>	Other R Clavicle surgery UCLH Prep 11am Out of recovery 5:30pm (woke u... Other More >>	Other Eve physio session (legs and hips only) Pain levels super high pos... C: 0:30:00	Custom Physio exercises 3-4 x per day (30 mins) C: 1:30:00	Custom Physio exercises 3-4 x per day (30 mins) + evening walk C: 1:30:00	Custom Physio exercises 3-4 x per day (30 mins) + evening walk C: 1:30:00		Completed	
							Total time	8:30:00	
							Custom Dur	7:30:00	
							Other Dur	1:00:00	
							Weekly Goals	More >>	
13	14	15	16	17	18	19	Aug 13 - Aug 19		
Custom Physio exercises 3-4 x per day (30 mins) + evening walk C: 1:30:00	Custom Physio exercises 3-4 x per day (30 mins) + evening walk C: 1:30:00	Other Fracture clinic app - Kingston hosp outpatients Custom Physio exercises 3-4 x per day (30 More >>	Other Hydro session Teddington pool C: 0:30:00 Custom Physio exercises 3-4 x per day (30 More >>	Custom Physio exercises 3-4 x per day (30 mins) + evening walk C: 1:30:00	Other Hydro session Teddington pool C: 0:30:00 Custom Physio exercises 3-4 x per day (30 More >>	Custom Physio exercises 3-4 x per day (30 mins) + evening walk C: 1:30:00		Completed	
							Total time	11:30:00	
							Custom Dur	10:30:00	
							Other Dur	1:00:00	
							Weekly Goals	More >>	
20	21	22	23	24	25	26	Aug 20 - Aug 26		
Custom Physio exercises 3-4 x per day (30 mins) + evening walk C: 1:30:00	Other Hydro session Teddington pool C: 0:30:00 Other Physio4Life - Catherine Cran More >>	Custom Physio exercises 3-4 x per day (30 mins) + evening walk C: 1:30:00	Other UCLH Fracture clinic app (Dad left for AUS) 2 WEEKS POST-SURGERY Custom More >>	Custom Physio exercises 3-4 x per day (30 mins) + evening walk C: 1:30:00	Other Hydro session Teddington pool C: 0:30:00 Custom Physio exercises 3-4 x per day (30 More >>	Custom Physio exercises 3-4 x per day (30 mins) + evening walk C: 1:30:00		Completed	
							Total time	11:00:00	
							Custom Dur	9:00:00	
							Other Dur	2:00:00	
							Weekly Goals	More >>	

I was ready to start increasing my water therapy to walking movement, with the hope that it would continue the good work on developing hip function, particularly on my right leg. Due to the attachments to the broken side of the pelvis, the right leg was noticeably weak and restricted. Lifting this leg took a lot of effort and connection through the middle of my core to protect my lower back and the diagonally opposite fracture site around the sacrum and lower back. I quickly learned how to avoid setting off a chain reaction with mindful, controlled movement and hoped there would be a day when I could move intuitively and automatically without pain concerns. Every day involved pain, stiffness and initiating uncomfortable movement in varying degrees. I'd forgotten what it was like to live pain free.

Finding ways to progress the healing process and regain movement range without pain led me to consider all of the benefits of aqua running. I'd used this as part of recovery on a regular basis when competing to great effect. I was very keen to see if the non-weight-bearing activity could help with strengthening the hip flexor from its damaged anchorage to my broken pelvis. This area was still quite distended and looked strangely asymmetrical compared with the left side. Not a good look!

My aim was to reproduce walking movement and continue working on range and strength in hip, back and leg movement using the resistance, warmth and pressure of the water. Having a small pool with varied depths nearby allowed me to independently access this type of session whenever I wanted. I started off with short sessions of 10 to 15 minutes supported with an aqua-running belt and moving in a walking-specific way.

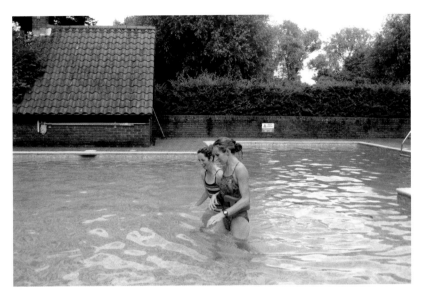

Aqua walking and running in deep water

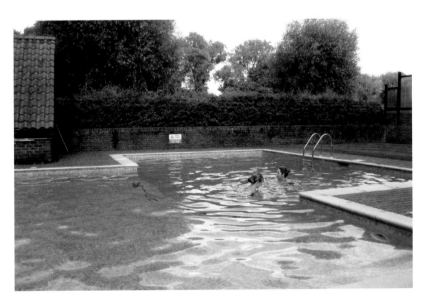

Use a flotation belt to support posture

Pool walking sessions:

What you need:

Flotation belt to support correct posture

Deep water area in a pool, at least 3 m x 2 m

Stopwatch or pool clock

How to do it:

1. Ensure the flotation belt fits closely around your waist.

2. Warm up with slow suspended walking movement in the deep water.

3. Aim to use your arms and legs in combination with each other, as diagonal pairs.

4. Keep your feet flat to replicate how you move on land.

5. Maintain upright posture and avoid leaning forward.

6. Engage hip flexors, glutes and hamstrings as you move the legs in large circular movements forwards.

7. Focus on quality of movement, not how far you travel. Distance over time is not important!

8. Work to leg cadence; count the number of revolutions your left or right leg makes over 60 seconds.

9. Aim to replicate brisk walking pace within a range of 50 to 70 spm (strides per minute).

10. Use an audible timing device or count your spm at regular intervals throughout your session.

When to progress:

Start with a session of 10 to 15 minutes two to three times per week.

Gradually increase the duration of sessions by 5 to 10 minutes per week as individual injury sites respond to mobilisation in water.

Structure the sessions as warm-up (50-60 spm), main set (60-70 spm) and cool-down (50-60 spm).

By exaggerating the range of movement in my legs the hip flexors, glutes, quads and hamstrings all had to engage. The problematic right hip flexor was always stiff but would become less painful as I walked in the deep water if I kept myself upright.

The two or three aqua walk sessions each week meant I was in a pool almost every day. I developed a series of rehab sessions with a warm-up, a focus on technique, rhythm and movement range and a cool-down. My legs always felt light and easier to move back on the land – the benefits were obvious. Rehab exercises after an aqua session were always less of a challenge, and my evening gait-focused walks progressed from grass to less forgiving hard footpaths. I used the sound of my footfall on the hard ground to make tiny adjustments to land more softly and with control.

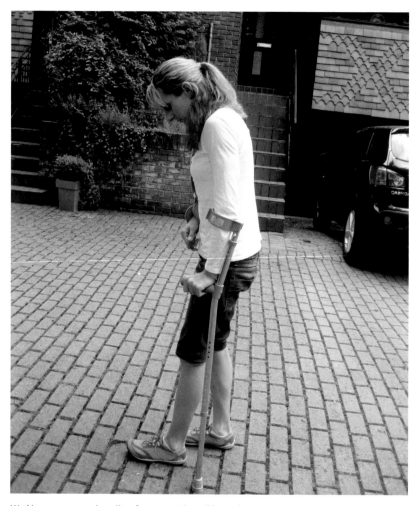

Working on range and quality of movement in walking gait

After three months I decided the time had come to wean myself off the painkillers. I was acutely aware that with the numbing effect of the drugs I was presented with a very nice picture of my pain management and recovery. I didn't want to rely on them any longer than I had to. What I wasn't sure of was the reality of life without the drugs.

I wanted to be more in tune with my body, but I recognised much of the effect of the medication was positive. I had never slept so much, and the high levels of fatigue encouraged me to rest often, which could only help the healing process.

I planned reducing my daily prescription of 400 mg of tramadol, 1200 mg of ibuprofen and 4000 mg of paracetemol. There was little advice to hand about how to go about this. It wasn't a topic for any of my outpatient appointments. My GP had not discussed the list of pain medication I was taking or how long I would be likely to require it.

The first week I noticed more pain and stiffness on waking. In the afternoons it took me a while to get movement quality going when I took my walk. On occasions when relaxing or asleep I found myself somehow forgetting to breathe and suddenly gasping for breath. It seemed that some of the automatic processes required for natural, normal breathing had been switched off by the medication.

The second week my sleep was disturbed with vivid dreams and flashbacks to the accident accompanied by night sweats. I felt emotionally flat during the day through lack of sleep. I had to make a concerted effort to accept invitations to be visited or to be with my friends at weekends.

During the day I experienced electrical tingling nerve impulses up and down my back. I could not sit at my desk or concentrate on any task for more than a few minutes. I was astounded at how restless I had become and by how ill I felt. At night I was wide awake, resorting to all-night 12-hour stints watching films, often the same ones over and over, in the hope this would induce sleep.

It was very difficult living alone, and I grew irrationally desperate, at one point I wanted to book a flight anywhere, just to get away.

I began to recognise through the haze that I was experiencing withdrawal symptoms from the morphine-like drug, tramadol. Occasionally I found myself thinking I needed to reinstate my dose of the yellow and green pills again to alleviate the symptoms.

Once I reached the fourth week and had researched common side effects of tramadol, I started to understand that the constant pain and crazy symptoms I was experiencing wasn't uncommon. It was a relief at this point to discover just how powerfully the drug worked.

I figured I was perhaps through the worst stages of withdrawal and dependency on the drug and had managed the process myself so decided it was best to dispose of the remaining tramadol medication, to remove the temptation to take it again.

After a few weeks I had adjusted to being in more pain than usual, less able to sleep having breathing difficulties, lack of appetite, restlessness and tingling in my spine and neck.

I focused on getting to hydrotherapy sessions, working through physical exercises at the usual times that I would take medication to help structure my day. Mornings were always difficult, and maintaining a daily dose of paracetamol helped relieve some of the feverish symptoms.

After eight weeks I started to feel a bit more like myself. I couldn't recall where most of September had gone. It was scary that four weeks of my life had simply disappeared.

Pain medication explained:

Opioid
A man-made drug with morphine-like action.

Mechanism of action of morphine
Morphine (and drugs which are synthetic opioids) produces its effects by binding to opioid receptors, which are found throughout the body. There are four types these receptors: μu, kappa, delta and OFQ/N receptors.

Activation of the μu receptors causes pain relief, mood alteration (euphoria and decreased anxiety), decreased gastrointestinal tract motility (causing constipation), decreased respiratory drive (causing death in overdose), nausea and vomiting, itching and pinpoint pupils.

Tolerance
When a patient takes opioids in reasonable doses for a relatively long period of time (e.g., 50-100 mg tramadol 4 times daily for over 10 days) the body begins to 'down regulate' its μu receptors. In other words, it begins to internalise them into the cell so that they are not available at the surface to be stimulated by the drug. This means that the same dose of drug will no longer produce the same effect in terms of pain relief.

On the positive side, some of the side effects will also decrease, although not the constipation or pinpoint pupils. In order, therefore, to maintain adequate pain relief, it can become necessary to increase the dose of drug. When people use morphine recreationally, seeking the high and euphoria of the drug, this is why they have to increase their consumption as time goes on.

Physical dependence

The continuous administration of opioids leads to physical dependence. This means that when the drug is stopped, physical withdrawal is experienced. This is because the μu receptors have been down-regulated, leaving fewer available to be stimulated by endogenously occurring opiates (i.e., the ones our bodies produce naturally), meaning the body cannot maintain its 'pre-opioid use' levels of stimulation.

Withdrawal

The symptoms of withdrawal include: diarrhoea, runny nose, sweating, tearing, hair standing on end (hence the phrase 'cold-turkey'), shivering, nausea and vomiting, anxiety, disordered sleep, restlessness, constant yawning, tremors, abdominal pain, muscle cramps and all over body pain and a craving for the medication.

Weaning off

Acknowledge that the process may be extremely difficult and unpleasant and may last for weeks to months. A sensible strategy is to do it slowly and not push on too quickly as this may ultimately result in greater success.

The timescale will vary depending on how long the patient has been on the medication, how high the dose has been and the effects the drug has on them. A range of bio-pycho-social factors will also come into play (e.g., social support, personality, individual coping strategies, etc.).

Tramadol has a second layer of problems in addition to its opioid effects because, as well as stimulating the μu receptor, it also acts as a noradrenaline-serotonin reuptake inhibitor. These are neurotransmitters released in the brain and heavily influence arousal and mood. Low levels of these neurotransmitters are implicated in depression and modern antidepressants act to increase their levels in the brain. For example, citalopram = selective serotonin reuptake inhibitor (SSRI) or venlafaxine = noradrenaline serotonin reuptake inhibitor (NSRI).

An increase in these chemicals can be helpful not only for depression, but also for neuropathic (nerve) pain and so the way in which tramadol modulates these chemicals makes it a very effective pain killer. However, it can make coming off tramadol an even more difficult experience, as it is akin to coming off morphine and an antidepressant at the same time. Additional symptoms of tramadol withdrawal attributable to the NSRI effect include anxiety, depression, severe mood swings, 'brain zaps' (sensation of electric shocks), vivid dreams, headaches, flu-like symptoms and insomnia, amongst others.

Kate McCombe, *consultant anaesthetist, Frimley Park Hospital*

Suggested Weaning Program:

From a starting dose of 100 mg tramadol 4x per day:

Week 1: Reduce 50 mg from one of the 4x daily doses.
Week 2: Reduce 50 mg from another of the 4x daily doses. Take 100 mg morning and night.
Week 3: Take 50 mg 3x day, 100 mg once per day (at night).
Week 4: 50 mg 4x per day.
Week 5: 50 mg 3x per day.
Week 6: 50 mg 2x per day.
Week 7: 50 mg only at night.
Week 8: 50 mg on alternate nights.
Week 9: Stop.

Aim to make a decrease in dose once a week, but if this gets too tough to do, back up then try again after another week and if necessary spend two weeks on a step.

Take regular paracetamol 4x per day if required to manage muscle aches, pains and feverish symptoms.

Example of weaning program (numbers below represent mg of tramadol to be taken at 6:00 12:00 18:00 22:00-00:00 depending on bedtime):

100 50 100 100
100 50 50 100
50 50 50 100
50 50 50 50
50 50 50
50 50
50 just at night
50 on alternate nights
Stop

If it becomes challenging:

» Seek help from the GP

» Simple analgesics such as paracetamol and ibuprofen may help with the muscle pains.

» Immodium may help with diarrhoea.

» If anxiety/sleeplessness are a problem, the GP may prescribe a short course of sleeping tablets (benzodiazepines, diazepam); however, these also cause physical dependence and addiction and so should only be taken for short periods of time.

» Alternatively use diphenhydramine (Nytol) or Nytol herbal to promote sleeping patterns. Some patients find aromatherapy or massage can help with relaxation to reduce anxiety and sleep. Good nutrition, hydration and routine and good sleep hygiene also help.

» Chewing sugar-free gum can help with the dry mouth.

» Domperidone melts are available over the counter (motilium), which can help with nausea.

» A drug called pregabalin can be prescribed for ongoing neuropathic (nerve) pain. This has the effect of manipulating serotonin, which is good for this type of pain, without the opioid effect. It also helps to improve anxiety has the added bonus of improving stage 2 sleep.

Karin Cannons, *nurse consultant in Pain Management at Frimley Park Hospital*

Monday 1 October 2012

The police and my solicitor informed me of this being the Crown Prosecution Service court date for the driver who caused my injuries. He was found guilty of driving without due care and attention. I was surprised to learn that he appealed the charge, and the case would be heard again in a few weeks. It was hard not to let this news not have a negative impact on my recovery.

While I was struggling to find any semblance of normality and independence in daily life, it was difficult to understand his lack of responsibility for being unable to follow the rules of the road and causing my life-changing injuries. I was lucky to have survived by not crashing into or over his car. My life had been significantly changed. Although I tried, I couldn't help wondering how he could justify his actions to his granddaughter and wife who were in his car at the time he caused the accident.

I started working with a Cognitive Behavioural Therapist. The dawning realisation that I was struggling to cope with rebuilding my life was brought sharply into focus in the harsh reality of daily life without powerful opioid pain medication. I was no longer was wearing rose-coloured glasses to view the world and needed expert help to understand how I would tackle the longer process of readjustment to my completely different life.

Further to the adjustment, I was becoming anxious over my recovery, worrying about my financial situation and unable to bear thinking about the longer-term impact on my life. Coming off the pain medication highlighted the daily concentration issues, flashbacks to the accident and sleep disruption. I avoided public places and going out and socializing with friends, and I wanted to stop the downward spiral. Reluctantly I went back to the GP to ask for help.

I was referred to a CBT (Cognitive Behaviour Therapy) Specialist Counsellor. Her initial assessment determined that I required intervention and treatment as a result of the accident trauma and after effects, with the aim to reduce the symptoms of PTS (Post-Traumatic Stress).

A series of weekly appointments worked through a process of making sense of what had happened and understanding triggers that provoked sensitivity, avoidance or unexpected reactions. Having a structured approach to consciously work through a process helped me synthesise the feedback overload that happened in an instant at the accident scene. Over the three months I learned to recognise and apply different behavioural techniques to control fear and anxiety.

A 'go-to' for therapy:

Post-Traumatic Stress Disorder (PTSD)
Is an anxiety disorder caused by very stressful, frightening or distressing events, such as a serious road accident.

Is estimated to affect 1 in every 3 people who have a traumatic experience.

Can develop immediately after someone experiences a disturbing event or can occur weeks, months or even years later.

Symptoms include reliving the event through nightmares and flashbacks or experiencing feelings of isolation, irritability and guilt.

Sleeping issues are commonly experienced, as are concentration issues significantly impacting on the person's daily life.

PTSD can be successfully treated with watchful waiting, psychological treatment such as cognitive behavioural therapy (CBT) eye movement desensitisation and reprocessing (EMDR) or antidepressant medication.

Cognitive Behaviour Therapy (CBT)
Talking therapy aiming to break overwhelming problem down into parts.

Develops ways to change the negative patterns to make sense of the trauma.

Aims to identify practical ways of dealing with problems and issues after a traumatic event.

Gain control of fear and distress through behavioural experiments.

Homework exercises are used to practice applying different thought patterns to find solutions.

Encouragement to gradually restart activities if avoiding after traumatic experience.

I was keen to introduce swimming to my rehabilitation program once the physiotherapist gave me the go-ahead that I could rotate the shoulder and arm. During the eight weeks following shoulder surgery a new set of exercises had been introduced to my rehab. Initial exercises had me moving the arm and hand gently each day, limited to below shoulder height. This became more functional over the weeks as I could start to extend the range of movement with my right arm upwards of my shoulder for the first time since the accident.

My shoulder and right arm was weak and lacked co-ordination initially, and a daily regimen of movement was required before contemplating swimming again. Much of the shoulder and upper arm felt numb to touch due to the nerve block from surgery. Introducing some tactile manipulation regularly when in hydrotherapy sessions and using the warm environment to stimulate the nerve endings I hoped might improve the sensory feedback.

The best place to start swimming was from a point of re-establishing some feel for the water, using sculling drills and a pull buoy to keep my hips elevated. This initially reduced the amount of strain on my lower back or hips by reducing the tendency to kick the legs for buoyancy or to remain close to the surface. Moving into deep water for the first time was a slightly surreal experience. I had to take a leap of faith. I wasn't entirely convinced I wouldn't sink. I didn't. Miraculously I found myself reasonably buoyant despite perceiving I lacked co-ordination. Once I could support myself in the water horizontally without any back strain or pain, light kicking was introduced with fins whilst sculling. By swimming repeats across the pool with rest intervals as needed, I composed a short 10- to 15-minute technique session.

The initial sessions were limited to time rather than distance. It was hard to contemplate that a 3- to 4-kilometre session in an hour used to be a 'normal' training swim for me. A short, technical session of 10 minutes was a challenge to begin with. After a few sessions I could feel the water and the gentle mobility on the body supported by training aids such as fins and a pull buoy had a dynamic stretching affect on the hip flexors, shoulders, spine and hamstrings.

Trying to introduce freestyle with full rotation through the shoulders and recovering the arms above the water was put off for a few weeks until I had my feel for the water back. My arms felt heavy and without purpose or co-ordination. I completed one to two swim sessions each week, alternating drills and kicking with fins to gradually build up my time in the water to 20 minutes.

After a number of sessions and, accompanied by a friend on my first 'swim', I tried freestyle for a few strokes. It was disjointed and awkward with the right shoulder feeling uncomfortable and restricted and, my right arm heavy, hard to lift and unco-ordinated over the top of the water.

A short distance later I had managed to string together a stroke of sorts with a little recovery in between. I recognised that both rotation from my hip and back injuries as well as limited shoulder range was causing the effects I could feel and that were observed while I tried to swim. I was nevertheless very happy at my success in achieving 10 metres of freestyle; it was another great achievement.

Saturday 13 October 2012

Returning to the masters training sessions was a significant breakthrough morning in October. I completed just half the session, as my progression had been to 30 minutes in the pool sessions I had been completing on my own. I was overcome to receive a round of applause from all of the swimmers as I rejoined my old lane, just four months after my accident. I was still sporting the faded branding on my right hip and back and was acutely aware of how vulnerable my shoulder, back and hips felt as other swimmers passed.

Occasionally I would stop and move out of the way of a perceived collision in the medley sets. Adam, the coach, was excellent at differentiating the session plan for me, unhesitatingly recommending that I complete freestyle or again assisted kicking drills if the sessions demanded medley or fast-paced efforts.

I was thoroughly exhausted and sore all over after the first session but elated to have overcome my fears and doubts. I celebrated with a hydro session immediately afterwards to counteract any increase in pain levels for the first few weeks after rejoining the masters Saturday morning swim. I was back!

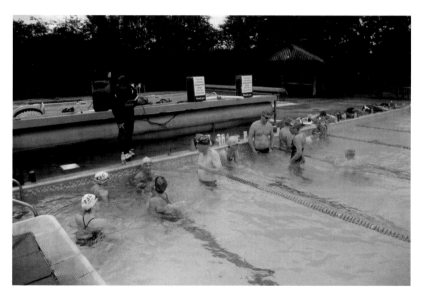

It's a significant confidence boost for the athlete to rejoin group sessions, particularly if the coach provides differentiation for the initial sessions to assist the transition from pre-training to full training.

Tuesday 13 November 2012

Progressing my rehabilitation to the next stage with the help of a specialist physical trainer was the next main breakthrough. Working through rehabilitation exercises and physio every day it was obvious in the five months since the accident that I needed to regain muscular strength to facilitate the links between function and my previous sports.

I started weekly strength and conditioning sessions with a focus on form, monitoring how my back and spine stabilised through a series of progressive loading exercises. A significant emphasis on core control was necessary from the early stages, and it was surprising how difficult the smallest range of movement quickly felt unsupported. Many exercises focused also on balance and stabilisation through the legs and hips, as my right leg was limited in range compared with the left. It was also sore on a regular basis throughout the week, as a result of increasing my mobility and time on legs working and beginning to carry light items around.

The strength sessions helped to functionally prepare the body for increasingly more independent and working life, with the overall aim to transition back into swimming, cycling and eventually running. I saw it as a long-term project and enjoyed being back in the gym again. Even though all of the exercises seemed very basic, I could feel how beneficial they were afterwards and struggled to do them initially on my own after the guided sessions with the trainer, Bruce.

At the six-month stage post accident I made arrangements to streamline my physiotherapy appointments and process for time efficiency. Having multiple appointments at different practices was detracting massively from the practicalities of trying to re-establish my business and coaching activities. From a recovery perspective I sought a more holistic, functional, whole-body approach and decided to self-fund private sessions with one physiotherapist.

It was immediately obvious this was a good decision. With a single appointment each week and the same therapist for continuity, a systematic approach was undertaken to work through the combined and separate issues prevailing from a high-speed accident. The knock-on effects to other areas of the body, compensation in unexpected ways and varied recovery times for each injury site all had to be factored in and reviewed as a whole rather than parts. Since weaning off the high levels of pain medication I had become aware of new aches and pains, including an area behind my shoulder blades. It was highlighted when I returned to swimming and tried to rotate left and right with an arm extended, and I had difficulty breathing deeply, twisting or lifting on one side.

I visited my GP three times over a number of weeks but was told it was just a soft tissue injury which would go away. It didn't. In the end my physiotherapist assessed the area and confirmed there seemed to be a problem with the rib and possibly some vertebrae. I went back to the doctor and was referred for a chest X-ray and MRI scan of the thoracic spine.

I only had a limited number of sessions with the physio, and I was keen to utilise them well. Each week I left with a more comprehensive set of exercises to build upon and progress. This enhanced the strength and conditioning work I was undertaking with Bruce in the gym and provided a more joined-up approach to the rehab process.

Weekly rehab plan, 2-3 months:
Stage 1 – mobility and physiotherapy

Monday: physio exercises for 30 min am/pm, walk 20 min

Tuesday: physio exercises (am/pm), hydro session 30 min

Wednesday: physio exercises (am/pm), walk 20 min

Thursday: physio exercises am/pm, walk 20 min

Physio session

Friday: physio exercises am/pm, walk 20 min

Saturday: physio exercises am/pm, hydro session 30 min

Sunday: physio exercises, yoga 30-45 min, walk 30-60 min

Weekly rehab, 5-6 months:
Stage 2 – function and strength

Monday: physio exercises 30 min am/pm, swim session 40-50 min

Tuesday: strength and conditioning session 30-45 min, walk 30-60 min

Wednesday: physio exercises, indoor bike/turbo session 30 min

Thursday: strength and conditioning session 30-45 min, swim session 40-50 min

Friday: physio exercises 30 min am/pm, yoga session 45-60 min

Saturday: swim session 60 min, hydro session 30 min

Sunday: long walk 60-90 min, yoga 60-75 min

Weekly rehab, 10-12 months:
Stage 3 – transition into multisport

Tuesday 27 November 2012

My counselling appointments each week had been going well. Each week I had a homework exercise to complete and if possible implement, which almost immediately started to change the way I felt. The sessions also helped me to recognise that I needed to work on getting back onto a bike again. I wasn't sure I could physically manage perching on a bike saddle, as sitting on a hard surface or chair wasn't an option at this stage of my recovery. It would have to be a padded seat!

I researched many different saddles on the market, tried all of the options I had at home on a stationary bike indoors on the turbo trainer and bought a padded saddle cover. I could not find a solution that would allow me to sit on a bike saddle for more than a few minutes without excruciating pain from my pelvis fracture site. Having a bike in my living room set up on a turbo trainer was not by choice; it was a necessary part of my recovery to view it regularly and accept it as it was before the accident.

It took a number of weeks to become desensitised to the view of a bike ready for me to ride and train on again. I eventually abandoned my own bike in favour of the gym indoor bike. I discovered I could sit on a gym bike's more comfortable saddle for up to 10 minutes. It was a more upright position that assisted my lower back compared with my road bike. This was the breakthrough discovery I needed to start the process of pushing the pedals again.

Once I started the process of training on the bike again, I could look to replicate the comfort on a road bike setup. It would involve building a new bike! This was one of my favourite projects I would typically plan early in the New Year as I received my sponsored bikes each season. It felt familiar territory. However, I would need to ask the questions of my recovering injuries and body on a weekly basis until I could cycle for 30 minutes. This seemed a huge task at this stage, much like walking unassisted by the elbow crutch for the first time. Another mountain to climb.

Starting to plan progression was a familiar process, and I started to believe that I could start to prepare for next summer's Alps training weeks. All I needed was time to gain my confidence back on the bike and coax my injuries to keep mending and repairing at a similar rate in the next six months. I did not want to let down the group of clients already booked on the summer cycle trip. The week involved cycling 14 mountain passes over the classic 'Route des Grandes Alpes' from Geneva to Nice, 650 kilometres in total.

Committing to the process of maintaining a continued existence outside my comfort zone seemed the most logical, important and daunting step. How would I ever manage to cycle six to eight hours a day for a week leading a group of cyclists over the northern and southern Alps? I couldn't even sit without pain for 5 minutes on an indoor static bike. The first step was to find a way and start working out a plan.

'Outside your comfort zone, you will find the extraordinary.'

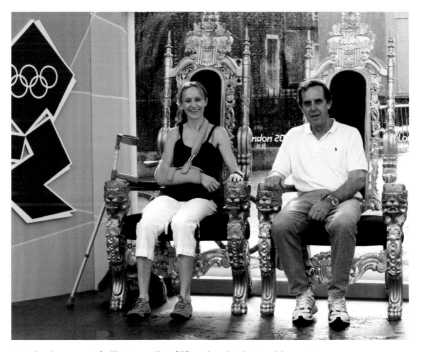

Functional movement facilitates quality of life and motivation to rejoin sport.

CHAPTER 7:
STAGED REHABILITATION

Biggest achievement: Cycling for 2-4 hours with only moderate level discomfort

Elevation gain: 235 m
Distance: 110 km

December 2012

I grew to appreciate the positive effect of warm temperatures on my injuries as the winter months set in. Swim training outdoors on a Saturday morning with the masters followed by a hydrotherapy session proved useful in offsetting the aftereffects of exercising compounded by being outside in cold temperatures.

My lower back would always be tight and painful in any range after a session in the pool, making walking, picking things up and carrying bags a problem. Everything had to be completed slowly for the remainder of the day until the muscle tension released and relaxed. Heat and warmth helped immensely, and I used an infrared lamp on specific areas that continued to be painful into the evening before sleeping.

There was a definite connection between warmth and pain relief and increased range of movement. I researched the impact of warm temperature climates, increased vitamin D production from exposure to sunlight on bone healing and accelerated recovery.

From skiers to runners to swimmers, athletes recovering from serious injuries headed somewhere warm to recover. It was a common theme. I decided to spend four weeks in the southern hemisphere's warmer climates.

It made sense to attempt the long haul flight to Australia in two parts. I would stop for a week's rest in Thailand on the way to spend Christmas with my family in Sydney. I looked forward to celebrating the end of a tough year with some downtime away from the daily struggles of rebuilding my body and business.

The flight was a long haul with luggage, however, and was no easy task. I used to enjoy travelling to international races – heavy bag and bike in tow. Now, I quickly realised my injury limitations, even with just one bag. A fit and strong body was the missing part of the equation for solo international travel.

The metal plate in my shoulder frequently set off the security alarms on the pre-flight checks. Carrying even a light bag on my right shoulder was impossible due to the discomfort of the metal on skin. Dragging luggage was not an option either because of the problems with my lower back and pelvis. A trolley was a good solution. The flights left me with a significant amount of back pain, and after hours on the plane finding a comfortable position to sit in was impossible.

I arrived at the beachfront resort north of Phuket after 24 hours travelling and was more than ready for a week of recuperation.

Tips for travelling long distance with injuries:

Choose lightweight, easy-to-manoeuvre luggage.

Pack as light as possible.

Taxi!

Seek advice from GP before flight and source pain medication and analgesics in case you need them on long-haul flights.

If you intend to book an exit seat for more space, if not in premium economy, business or first class, ensure you meet the mobility requirements.

Keep hydrated during the flight.

Move from your seat every 60 to 90 minutes to move and stretch.

Book the most optimal connecting flights involving the least transit between terminals with luggage if not checked all the way through.

Have a letter from your surgeon or GP regarding any metalwork as a result of injuries (non-EU countries).

Plan a recovery day for the first 24 hours after arrival.

A beach holiday with one of my best friends was perfect reward for getting through the previous six months. Waking up the first morning highlighted just how challenging the long journey getting to Asia had been for my injuries. It was a pleasant change to have constantly warm temperatures all day, and I was confident that it would prove to be a perfect environment for recovery. Debbie and I had been friends since primary school, and we had plenty of catching up to do.

Over the week we made the most of fresh nutritious meals prepared daily, numerous options for water-based sessions, consistently warm daily temperatures and the sunshine. To my delight and relief my range of movement around injury sites was enhanced, pain levels reduced and I slept well. I had a huge, comfortable bed and used the pillow-under-the-knees trick to relieve pressure from my lower back.

The early morning sunrise beach yoga was a great way to start each day, checking in with the level of overnight injury stiffness, stretching from head to toe, working through gentle spinal twists and body-weight supported range of movement.

Having kilometres of pristine sandy beach to walk each day tempted me to take my first exploratory running strides. I had been wondering whether I could run again for many months.

It was a completely amazing but also quite scary feeling to engage my legs, balance, co-ordination and strength and lift myself into a run on soft sand for the first time in six months. I could hardly believe it at first.

Every day I looked forward to working through running-specific strength and rehabilitation exercises during my daily walk. Active engagement and drills seemed a logical progression to apply into running strides. It was like a bridge I had built from rehab into pre-training.

I was a long, long way from being able to resume training as I once knew it. I rarely contemplated how long that might take or even if it would be possible. By focusing on the present I was encouraged every day to seek increments of progress and enjoyed the process of rebuilding a new version of my physical self.

My running drills and technique sessions must have looked like comedy walking to anyone who happened to be on the beach. The exercises were very similar to running drills on the track before a speed session; however, I completed them in super slow motion. My aims were to improve co-ordination, movement patterns and functional strength. I could feel the neuromuscular patterns improving each time I lifted into a jog for a short stretch. My right leg and hip flexor felt disjointed, painful and awkward and took some convincing to engage. I celebrated a massive leap in progression to achieve a 'run' on the forgiving beach sand in Thailand.

Walking was the best rehabilitation for my injuries. This had gradually progressed from 20 minutes to an hour or more at home in the UK. On holiday I changed my walking plan up a little, with enhanced recovery management in a spa hotel. Alternate days I would perform a simple sequence of 50 run strides followed by 50 walking steps, repeated through five times. The other days I would simply walk for a few hours up the beach and then back again. The soft sand allowed me to assess my footfall, stride and imprint. I noticed the right footprint looked deeper and more pronounced than the left. This led to greater awareness when walking to understand how the the legs were moving differently.

Each day I would also be in the gym, replicating the strength and conditioning sessions I was used to completing at home. It was a perfect place for a break, with the spa facilities, water sports centre, beach and choice of Thai food. Each day I booked into the spa for a therapeutic massage to improve circulation or to spend time alternating warm and cold spa pools. My body felt better and better every day, and I noticed my back pain was easing.

Stand-up paddle boarding up and down the beachfront on the calm ocean was one of my favourite afternoon activities, despite being quite one-sided at paddling. Significant core stabilisation was needed to stay on the board, and it was quite a challenge, albeit a nice one.

By the time I left for Sydney I was very pleased the plan had worked. I felt the most recovered I had done in the many months since the accident.

The three weeks in Sydney over Christmas was great. It was nice to spend time with my family and friends, without distractions of work and running the business. I lapped up the sun and temperatures, feeling the repair and energy-giving benefits. I rented a 4x4 to get to the gym each day, visit family and friends and carry out my swimming tour of some of Sydney's best and most beautiful 50-metre outdoor pools. I soon established a routine of strength and conditioning, swimming and walking in my home town.

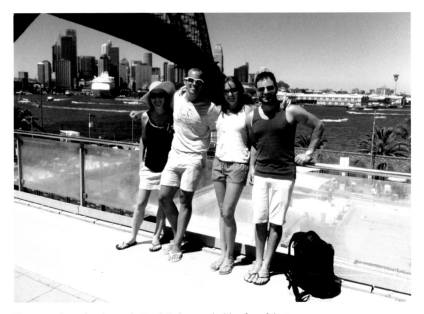

Warm-weather swimming at the North Sydney pool with a few of the team

Having the extra height and space in the car when getting in and out made a significant difference to my back and hip injuries. It was a lot more comfortable. The main problem with driving was occasional hypersensitivity to other drivers' sudden movements if they appeared quickly from my left side in a side road. The seatbelt also sat uncomfortably across the metal plate on my right clavicle.

I continued my daily focus on moving my body with the broader aim of linking back into my sports of swimming, cycling and running. The local gym I had used for years at university offered me temporary membership for three weeks. I enjoyed being in a familiar environment each day to swim, do my strength training in the gym and work out on the indoor bikes.

I worked with another experienced trainer who had links to the area I lived in Twickenham from his professional rugby days in England. He added some new perspectives to my strength training and monitored new movement patterns as I established them in sessions.

I made an appointment with a physiotherapist who was recommended by a good family friend. It provided another breakthrough. He assessed my injuries and provided strong encouragement for being able to return to running. I explained my progress so far and my first few 'runs' on the beach, which he endorsed. His opinion was that I could run again, as the major healing had been completed at the fracture sites of the various injuries.

It was a challenge mastering the progressive core and stability exercises during the session. An ultrasound on my deeper core muscles as I performed the exercises highlighted just how much more work needed to be done to rebalance and stabilise, particularly the injured side of my pelvis. I could barely manage to activate my core muscles while passively lying on the physio table.

Much more strength needed to be established before making the gradual transition back into multisport training.

The prospect of working through the 'return to jog' programme I hoped would reconnect some of the flow in movement that was lacking in my first few tentative runs on the beach. I was content to build from the ground back up again, if need be. I certainly did not feel that I was running inside the same body on any of my first few runs. It was all completely new and different, but it did not worry me that it would take time to re-establish. That I could potentially consider running again so soon was the best news I could get at Christmas. It felt as though I had only just started to walk a short time ago.

Applying the athlete mindset:

Understanding – recovery time is dependent on lifestyle factors, quality of nutrition and amount of sleep.

Knowledge – progress is not expected to be linear.

Patience – adaptation takes time.

There are no shortcuts!

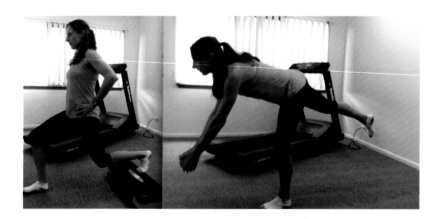

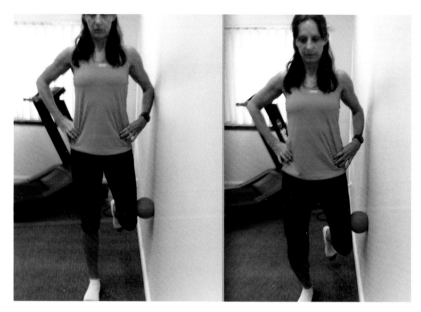

Physiotherapy exercises working on movement range, balance and strength for running

Return to jog programme – Phase 1

Level 0:

Build up to walking for 20 minutes at a comfortable speed.

Progress your speed towards 6.5 kph.

Once you can do this without aggravation or pain, then you can progress to the next level.

Level 1:

Day 1: Walk 4 minutes, Jog 1 minute, Walk 4 minutes and so on for 20 minutes.

Day 2: Rest/Weights/Swim/Cycle

Day 3: Walk 4 minutes/Jog 1 minute for 20 minutes

Day 4: Rest/Weights/Swim/Cycle

Progress to level 2 when level 1 causes no aggravation or pain during or after session.

Level 2:

Day 5: Walk 3 minutes/Jog 2 minutes or 3.5/1.5 minutes for 20 minutes

Day 6: Rest/Weights/Swim/Cycle

Day 7: Walk 3 minutes/Jog 2 minutes or 3.5/1.5 minutes for 20 minutes

Day 8: Rest/Weights/Swim/Cycle

Progress to level 3 when level 2 causes no aggravation or pain during or after session.

Level 3:

Day 9: Walk 2 minutes/Jog 3 minutes for 20 minutes

Day 10: Rest/Weights/Swim/Cycle

Day 11: Walk 2 minutes/Jog 3 minutes for 20 minutes

Day 12: Rest/Weights/Swim/Cycle

Progress to level 4 when level 3 causes no aggravation or pain during or after session.

Level 4:

Day 13: Walk 1 minute/Jog 4 minutes for 20 minutes

Day 14: Rest/Weights/Swim/Cycle

Day 15: Walk 1 minute/Jog 4 minutes for 20 minutes

Day 16: Rest/Weights/Swim/Cycle

Progress to level 5 when level 4 causes no aggravation or pain during or after session.

Level 5:

Day 17: Jog 20 minutes

Day 18: Rest/Weights/Swim/Cycle

Day 19: Jog 20 minutes

Day 20: Rest/Weights/Swim/Cycle

Level 6:

Review progress with your physiotherapist to progress to phase 2.

Oliver Weber, *titled sports physiotherapist, PhysioPoint Springwood, NSW Australia*

January 2013 – Bike rehab

Returning to London in January was a shock. The contrast of the month away in warm weather with my family and friends that had put a lot of the difficulties I'd overcome behind me left me feeling unsettled on my return. This was compounded by the results of the MRI scan on my upper back and neck. A fractured seventh thoracic vertebrae and 'wear and tear' damage to some of my neck vertebrae had been discovered on the scan. At least this explained why I had difficulties breathing, lying on my back, carrying heavy items and twisting through my back.

It was regarded as such low importance that an appointment to discuss the results was not deemed necessary, as no treatment was required. The fracture was apparently 'old' and not affecting the spinal column in any way. With a diagnosis I again reverted to self-managing the painful area with an infrared heat lamp and funding a private physiotherapist with experience in my injuries. He manipulated my spine with a manual release technique. Having my back and neck 'clicked' to release meant that the pain relief after his sessions was remarkable.

I did not know whether to carry on pushing to build my business back up or start looking for a full-time job. To get my business fully back up and running I would need to work day, night and weekends. It would require huge levels of energy, and there was no guarantee of success. It was a daunting prospect. It was a tough decision.

My first appointment was to see the counsellor I had been working with before I left for Australia. I had decided to maintain commitment to the process of trying to get my working and athletic life back on track.

Before I attended CBT sessions I had accepted my injuries were likely to prevent me from conducting my usual triathlon and cycling training activities, including working in the French Alps every summer. Having an experienced CBT therapist helped me to learn and apply CBT techniques to manage the disruption to all aspects of life post accident. Nancy was another person who like Debbie from the accident scene helped me immeasurably at a crucial time.

Tuesday 15 January 2013

I had spent some time planning how to progress back onto a bike outside. My indoor cycling sessions had increased to almost an hour with tolerable back and hip pain levels at aerobic intensity.

I decided a mountain bike would be key to making the leap from the safe indoor environment to the traffic-ridden road. Each stage of the return-to-bike process focused on a different aspect. The objective of this phase was to usefully transport me to my final therapy appointment, off the roads away from traffic.

I planned a route along the towpath by the river, a rough path on flat terrain. After the first five minutes, however, my injuries were being jolted around, and I was in serious pain. Having committed to the process and not wanting to be late, I pushed on, skirting any rougher parts of the path, potholes and ruts in favour of smoother surfaces. I was very relieved to pop on to some tarmac for the final 10 minutes of the 30-minute commute.

Pain aside, I enjoyed being back outside on the bike, connecting with the elements. Surprisingly I felt like I had not been off the bike at all. Nancy couldn't believe her eyes when she spotted me arriving on the bike. By the time I had secured my bike, she had come to meet me at the entrance door. It was a tearful start to the session. She was very proud of what I had achieved, and I was grateful for her support and the encouragement that let me believe I could overcome the fear and pain.

I had come so far in less than six months. I was back on the bike with a plan to help me overcome my fear. The treatment to make sense of the traumatic events with specific rationalisation on each area had worked. It symbolised the toughest and first step of any long mountain climb.

Bike rehabilitation plan:

Stage 1

Indoors on stationary trainer and bike or gym bike.

Short sessions starting with pain free or very low pain duration (10 minutes).

Aerobic intensity, easy effort.

Focus on symmetry in pedal strokes, rhythm and cadence.

Allow ample time for the injury sites to adapt before increasing duration.

Pain management post session – hydrotherapy, massage, stretching.

Physiotherapy for support – functional exercise and physical manipulation.

Start with 2-3 sessions per week.

Remain in stage 1 for at least 8 weeks depending on severity of injuries.

Stage 2

Indoors on trainer or outside on road or mountain bike.

Increase duration up to 60 minutes.

Aerobic intensity introducing short duration, moderate tempo efforts (sub threshold).

Focus on strength and endurance, hill-climbing technique using body weight to stand on lower cadence efforts.

Increase duration at a rate of <10% per week.

Pain management post session – hydrotherapy, massage, stretching, swimming, yoga.

Physiotherapy for support – functional exercise and physical manipulation.

Complete 3-5 sessions per week.

Continue with stage 2 for 2-6 months depending on adaptation and recovery.

Planning a return to outdoor cycling on my road bike rapidly highlighted my injury limitations due to back and hip pain. A simple two-minute spin revealed just how unsuitable my current road bike would be for rehabilitation. I took all of my bikes indoors one weekend and experimented on the stationary (turbo) trainer with different setups in attempt to identify a sustainable position, without success.

I was limited to a few minutes before the pain would become excruciating, and I would have to get off the bike. The indoor gym bikes were the most suitable option for all of the early (stage 1) rehabilitation work in the first three months because of the more relaxed setup and even weight distribution across the wider saddles. It also proved to be very effective option as I felt safe indoors, and it was easy to maintain constant effort, observe variation in power, pedal cycle and cadence.

Once I established a start point from 10 minutes in duration, I planned a conservative progression of sessions to complete two to three times a week. Having a plan to follow helped me commit to completing the sessions each week, with the realisation that I might be able to eventually cycle for an hour in a relatively manageable pain state.

The issue of returning to the road at some point was delayed until the spring months when it would be more realistic from the perspective of progression and weather conditions.

During the 8 to 12 weeks I gradually increased my cycling to 45 minutes and noticed a number of significant adaptations. The gradual increase in duration was manageable with weekly increments of 2 to 5 minutes. A conservative approach to training progression helped manage the reaction from the injuries with hydrotherapy or sports massage afterwards.

I experienced no setbacks during this early phase to return to cycling. During the sessions I varied my position more predominantly upright interspersed with short efforts in a more aerodynamic forward lean to stretch out more like my anticipated road bike setup. This proved no issues at the low intensity on an indoor bike. Distributing the weight through injury sites made immediate sense. Pedalling efficiency improved within the first week. The change was noticeable from odd-shaped pedalling feedback to smoother round circles using data from the static Wattbike. The neuromuscular patterning returned with the regularity of getting on the bike every other day.

It was remarkable how the body seemed to remember the activity. Positive progress throughout stage 1 led to researching a custom-built road bike that would replicate the positioning I had achieved indoors. I had found a reasonably comfortable position on a more upright gym bike. I also decided I needed a bike designed to absorb road vibration with optimal frame geometry and materials.

I eventually settled on sourcing a suitable road bike frame with Paris-Roubaix winning credentials. I reasoned this type of road bike would be both forgiving and lightweight. The long-term plan was to have a suitable bike spec for the Grand Alps tour, so it was built up with components to ensure it was a perfect climbing bike for the Alps. A number of different saddles were sourced and tried before a suitable solution was identified, none of my racing saddles were even remotely possible in a more adapted upright position. The weight distribution had to be distributed evenly as possible across a now asymmetrical area. This part of the process took the most persistence. I had to experiment and test as many options as possible. I wrote to saddle manufacturers to ask them for recommend options in their range for cyclists with my injuries. It took a long time to find a minimalistic mountain bike saddle in the end. It looked a little out of place on a racy carbon road bike but was the best solution.

Once the bike was built it looked fantastic and was lighter than any of my sponsored bikes had been. The final touch was a dynamic motion Retul fit to identify how the final setup would need to be adapted. The end result was a bike I could ride on the road. It provided the motivation for me to overcome the fears of being out in the traffic again.

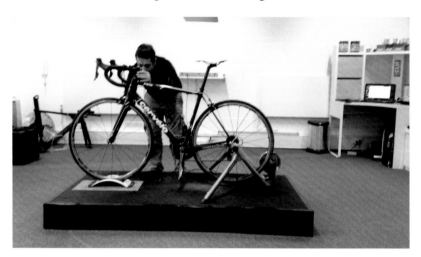

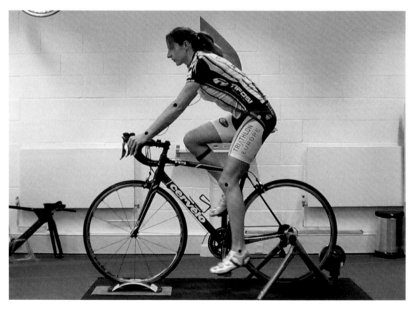

Retul fitting process using dynamic motion capture and flexibility assessment

My first few rides were at quiet traffic times in a closed park near to my home with my long-time training buddy Kerrie. It was great to be back on the road, and the bike fit and setup proved ideal to work from. I had to adapt to different positioning on the bike. I had a noticeable leg-length imbalance, and I was protecting my right side by curving my spine and body towards a slightly dropped right shoulder. It felt asymmetrical and awkward, and if static for too long fatigue set in.

My early sessions on the road were limited to an hour around the park – always accompanied. Kerrie intuitively rode on my right, shielding me from traffic which was hugely reassuring. I tended to overreact if cars appeared suddenly in front of us or from a side turning on my left. I hoped this hypersensitivity would subside over time.

I required more physio each week to manage the reactions from the multiple injury sites. As one area would subside, something else would flare up. Mainly I was in constant pain on and off the bike from where the fractures in my pelvis had healed. The saddle felt raised on one side because of the scar tissue that had built up. Physiotherapy sessions involved manual working of extremely painful scar tissue. The metal implement used resembled a levelled out ice cream scoop and was very effective over time, although barbaric to anyone who might have observed the process.

I recognised the need for time and patience over the winter months and planned the next progression into stage 2 with a trip to the smooth roads and renowned excellent cycling in Mallorca. It was exciting to look forward to a trip away, as a reward for the consistent effort since committing to the process to get back on the bike. The warmer weather cycling trip in a new environment that would not provide any reminders of the crash proved to be a breakthrough for cycling progression.

Over the week rides increased from two hours to four hours, always accompanied by my boyfriend. On our last day our ride distance totalled 100 kilometres, which seemed amazing. It was almost as though I had not had an injury which caused an extended break off the bike.

The smoother roads meant less vibration through my body, and the warmer conditions after the winter cycling at home led to significantly restored confidence levels. I felt at one with the bike again, settling into the rhythm of pedalling efficiently for hours with manageable pain after each session.

Again, pain management was key, and scheduling warm-weather therapy or massage and stretching after every session was by now a ritual I looked forward to. I chose a spa hotel with post-session recovery in mind. It was perfect!

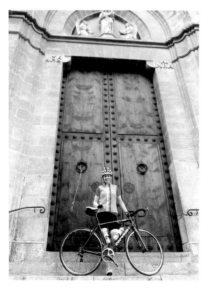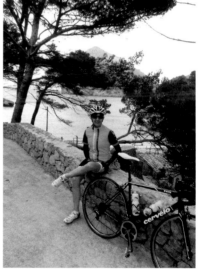

Getting back on the road in Mallorca

Top 10 tips for rehab:

1. Assess your requirements and progress weekly to develop your rehab plan and source further support proactively.

2. Both physical 'hands-on' physio and functional 'exercises-led' physiotherapy is often required at different stages of the process.

3. Anticipate additional requirements (e.g., physio, physical therapy, sports massage) to support or manage an incremental increase in exercise or pre-training.

4. Recognise and celebrate every breakthrough session, moment or new skill mastery.

5. Keep your goals in sight; keep moving towards them even if it is slowly.

6. Plan your progression; keep adjusting and adapting according to where you are right now, not where you want to be.

7. Refrain from loading up speed or intensity too quickly to avoid the 'boom and bust' training cycle.

8. Setbacks disrupt continuity and consistency. Avoid them.

9. Understand the body remembers previous movement patterning from your sport.

10. Investing a relatively modest amount in training hours will yield significantly large proportion of muscle memory being regained.

Table 3

STAGED RECOVERY PLAN TIMELINE MULTISPORT APPROACH
First 3-6 months: Swimming Hydrotherapy (water walking) Physiotherapy
6-12 months: Strength and conditioning Cycling Swimming Physiotherapy Yoga Pool rehab (water walking)
6-12 months onwards: Swimming Cycling strength and conditioning Yoga Physiotherapy Pool rehab (water running) Running

By spring my running had gradually progressed to a 20-minute continuous jog at a modest pace, following the return to jog programme. My cycling had been increasing as the weather improved; weekend rides were three to four hours and tolerable on good roads.

I had ridden past the accident site a few times and been overcome by emotion. The aftereffects had been managed with a forward focus on aspirations, as there were a number of nightmares, hypersensitive moments and flashbacks resulting from these outings.

The pain after sessions was managed reasonably well by spacing 'injury trigger' sessions in the week, interspersed with strength and conditioning, swimming and yoga. If in doubt another rest day and some physio or sports massage would need to be factored in. It was a challenge to co-ordinate, but I was finally in a place where I felt some of my athlete identity had been restored. I was training again, albeit at a different level, but the routine and reward was restored.

I had a new trusty steed that was a light, responsive and forgiving ride. New challenges lay ahead in the form of mountains!

Restoring athlete identity by transitioning from rehab into training:

Work with an experienced rehabilitation sports specialist for strength and conditioning sessions.

Ensure there is a plan in place, based on the quality of movement required for sports.

Monitor movement quality and athlete ability to repeat.

Aim for balanced range of movement, good patterning and fluency.

Once imbalances are identified, a sequence for reconstruction of complex movement patterns can be planned and practised with progression.

'Nature doesn't recognize good or bad, only balance or imbalance.'

Tremay Dobson, *elite running trainer, sports therapist and personal trainer*

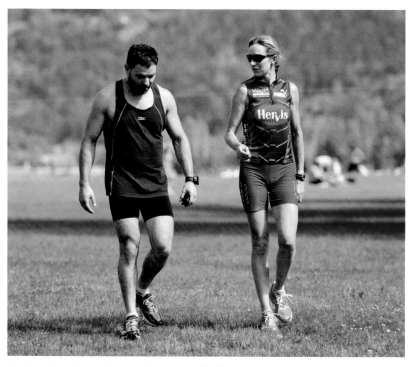

Coaching in the French Alps – triathlon race-specific bike-and-run session 2011

CHAPTER 8:
CLIMBING MOUNTAINS

Biggest achievement: Ascending 14 mountain passes[1], cycling the Route des Grandes Alpes from Geneva to the Mediterranean

Elevation gain: 13,720 m
Distance: 677 km

---

1   Mountain passes or 'cols': The lowest point of or saddle between two peaks, typically providing a pass from one side of a mountain range to another (Oxford English Dictionary)

Grand Alps tour

I returned from Mallorca with increased confidence to apply in my cycle training to improve aerobic and muscular endurance. With just three months before the summer I needed to avoid setbacks and maintain consistency in cycle training to take on the epic miles demanded by the Grand Alps tour. The ride itinerary had been tailored for the riders coming from Australia to include famous climbs such as Alpe D'Huez. I had vivid memories of the 21 switchbacks, having raced up the mountain in 2006 as my lead-up triathlon event to the ITU World Championships in 2006.

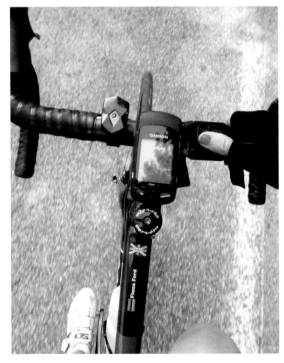

Successful alpine climbing requires consistent aerobic effort and pacing.

I hoped that my body would remember the endurance and strength required aerobically to ride consecutive days over the high Alps for a week. Seven years ago adopting a 'train hard, race easy' approach yielded extraordinary results where the demands of greater adaptation led to perfectly timed peak performance. I couldn't wait to be back immersed in my second home, the Alps, and fully focused on the organisation required for the group of Australian cyclists coming over for a once-in-a-lifetime trip cycling from Geneva to Nice over 17 mountain passes. This would be my third time over the Route des Grandes Alpes.

With just one cycle training week to organise, I wondered how I would ever be able to increase my workload back to my pre-injured capacity. Every summer I took for granted that I could organise, coach and oversee three to four triathlon and cycling weeks for up to two months with groups of various athletes coming out to France seeking a performance boost for races. I was fully stretched in resuming 40 to 50% of my coaching during the week, evenings and occasional weekends. Afternoon rests were required to ensure I could recover enough energy to coach my squad in the evenings. My income was vastly reduced, and outgoings to fund medical expenses and additional help had increased. I was strongly committed to keeping the business going and uncertain I could manage to work full-time at my present stage of recovery if the financial pressure became too great. Either way, I had to keep pushing on with my recovery as sensibly and swiftly as was physically possible. Survival provided strong motivation at the start of each day to push a sore and stiff body through yet another daily regime of movement.

My training had become more focused as a result of the goal to provide the cycling week in the Alps. The main components were cycling, strength and conditioning, swimming and some yoga. With most weeks leaving me exhausted and challenged to provide coaching activities, attend medical appointments and complete the physical work of rehabilitation, there was little point thinking too much further ahead.

I couldn't visualise exactly how my recovery and function would evolve in the months or even a year ahead. It was more efficient mentally and emotionally to focus on the day-to-day importance of where my recovery was at the present time. Managing my recovery within the next stage of rehabilitation back to sport required all my energy and focus. I was constantly reminded of how far I had come and how grateful I was to be back in training of sorts, albeit with a completely different purpose in mind. My friends and family were incredibly supportive and encouraging along all the steps of the process.

Be progressive!
Avoid the rehabilitation and training 'boom and bust' cycle.

How:
Begin with sessions at an 'unthreatening' level of difficulty.

Perform sport-specific movement at low intensity and speed until pain free.

Athlete should feel like he is going through the motions so he can focus entirely on his form.

Session support with training partners, coach or physio if required to monitor and provide feedback on quality of movement.

Review skills, judgement and awareness (e.g., clipping in and out of pedals, getting on and off the bike with new injury limitations).

Start to make connections to previous training routine and daily rhythm of challenging muscle groups followed by recovery.

Why:
Aiming to build from the ground back up helps avoid setbacks from pressure to return to sport too quickly.

Reinforces and re-establishes neural pathways over time.

Essential that form follows function, function follows form.

Continuity in strength and conditioning training will lessen chances of future injury or setbacks.

Improved confidence as strength and form continues to improve.

Heightened body awareness in movement has positive impact on sports performance in the long term.

Tania Cotton, *movement analyst, British chartered physiotherapist*

I enjoyed planning and working through my training progression. Even the smallest improvements were very motivating. The long endurance rides had gradually increased to three and four hours, with up to four sessions during the week predominantly aerobic intensity with a focus on hill climbing strength for sustained periods. I could feel myself getting stronger and recognised that aerobically I had not lost my foundation of fitness and conditioning. The engine just needed to be run at low to moderate intensity to bring about strength gains that muscle atrophy had taken away.

My injuries were getting more resilient to being constantly challenged in movement range and function. The long endurance rides were not overly demanding, and my time off the bike was spent on strength and conditioning work in the gym to increase power or stretching and aiming to achieve more symmetry and offset the obvious compensation from multiple injuries. It not a surprise to see how much atrophy had occurred, particularly in the lack of muscular shape of my legs, during the eight months after the accident. I didn't recognise my own strangely twisted body when I returned to yoga classes and was shocked to discover just how many limitations I now had to work around to gently coax the body back into a flexible state. There were many stretches I simply could not manage at first, and once I accepted this I could work from where I was, rather than think about what I used to be able to do.

Progressing from rehabilitation into running-specific training:

Firstly check the athlete's balance using static movements and co-ordination.

Example exercises: Plank, single-leg stand (eyes open, eyes closed), squad sit–stand

Select a series of strength and cardio exercises that will take the athlete from non-weight-bearing to partial weight-bearing to full weight-bearing exercises.

Example exercises:
Non-weight-bearing – Leg raises, wall angels, recumbent bike

Partial weight-bearing – Overhead squats, lateral band swings, upright bike

Full weight-bearing – Full squats, step-ups, lunges, running

More exercise progression would be incorporated as determined by the athlete.

Start off with a slow, deliberate process, gathering pace as the strength gains become evident.

Avoid regression by being thorough and not skipping parts of the process.

Continue consistently moving forwards and remember that as the injured leg (or area) grows stronger it may not necessarily grow in size.

Tremay Dobson, *elite running trainer, sports therapist and personal trainer*

The new bike was performing well, as light as a feather and absorbing much of the vibration on training rides. My confidence was improving; some rides I hardly thought about the prospect of falling from the bike again due to traffic or motorists. Still on certain days a simple trigger would set off a fearful chain of thoughts, and I would lose confidence. On these occasions, this was a terrible scenario. Riding with my training partner Kerrie and often many kilometres from home in the Surrey Hills I would have no alternative but to keep riding. As soon as I could control my emotions I would consciously take my mind off the negative thoughts and focus on something positive, anything!

An appreciation of being back on the bike, being able to pedal again and enjoying cycling for the freedom it brings would help me to manage the fear and symptoms. Having a great training partner was essential. If all else fails, simply following a wheel can provide immeasurable comfort and confidence.

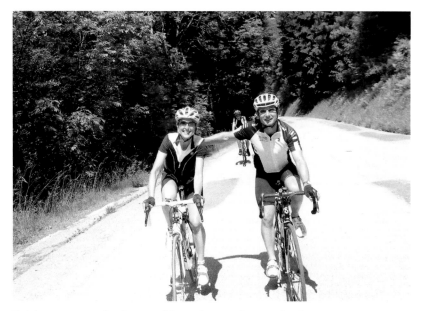

Training partners greatly enhance confidence when returning to road cycling.

Top tips for getting back on the bike – confidence-boosting progression:

Start indoors on a gym bike or stationary trainer.

Begin with short sessions up to 15 minutes.

Progress duration as pain stabilises or reduces during and after sessions.

Obtain a bike fit to identify limitations in range of movement through injury sites.

Optimise your existing bike setup if possible or custom spec a new build.

Source a bike frame that is designed to absorb road vibration, particularly if recovering from a back or hip injury.

177

Use the lightest and best quality components your budget will permit. They do make difference!

Identify suitable lightweight wheels with good quality hubs for the most efficient rolling ride.

Avoid stiff, heavy winter tyres.

Trial different saddles to identify a likely design to support your injuries. Think laterally and research mountain bike saddles and road and racing saddles that have similar designs.

Reduce the tyre pressure if you are cycle training on rough road surfaces to help absorb some of the impact through the bike to the body.

Fit powerful front and rear lights, including an integral camera (Fly6).

Source cushioned handlebar tape, particularly if recovering from shoulder injury.

Ride with a trusted training partner or small group to begin with; ensure they are well briefed if you require any specific considerations in traffic.

Accept the legacy of bike accident is heightened sense of fear and flashbacks for a period of time.

Factor some gradual exposure to anxiety triggers in training to develop confidence and a sense of dealing with adversity.

The first time I rode past the accident site was by chance, and I had little time to anticipate how I would react, such was the 'autopilot' state I was in when choosing the turning to lead us onto the fateful road. As I approached the junction I found it difficult not to look for the spot on the tarmac I had met at speed and lay broken, as if there would still be a mark or sign of the accident happening there nine months earlier. Passing the junction and breaking into a hot flush of sweaty emotion made it difficult to continue pedalling; all the energy had drained temporarily from my body.

Following the wheel that day, through tears, was the only option. I felt vulnerable and unsafe when cars came past or pulled out of side roads. On quiet roads I could enjoy my cycling, but I knew that becoming less sensitive to traffic was a part of the rebuilding process. Driving in my car past the accident site provoked similar emotions, and often these would provoke recurring dreams of lying injured in the middle of the road surrounded by traffic chaos.

Thankfully with each of the few occasions I rode past the junction, from all directions, there was less of an emotional response. Some days I simply opted not to ride or drive that way, if I anticipated there would be lots of traffic or simply didn't feel up to dealing with aftereffects like the flashbacks to the accident. One day my training group opted to ride from the side turning, approaching the junction the same way the driver's car would have. I stopped and unclipped safely at the side of the junction. Taking in the view helped me understand that the driver had not seen me, as he had not looked to his right before pulling out. This observation was verified and endorsed by the group I was riding with, before we rode on home. I felt angry with the driver for the first time.

In contrast to race-specific conditioning, I trained on a range of different bikes in sessions each week to utilise slightly different muscle groups and avoid overloading in particular my back, sacrum or pelvis. The degree of pain following each session was inevitably related to duration of sessions, and this was increased gradually over six months.

Physio sessions each week worked through a progression of manipulation and exercises at each injury site on a weekly basis. Which injury was on the weekly 'rota' directly correlated to the degree of pain in the days before the physio appointment. Scheduling a weekly sports massage to manage soft tissue and release tension in fascia significantly helped continued progression as inevitably areas would become stiff and sore as a result of training with so much compensation present from the multiple injury sites. It was a process that simply couldn't be rushed; patience was key. I had to adapt to different positioning on the bike, leg-length imbalance, curving of the spine towards the right, right shoulder rotated forwards and dropped and a general perception of asymmetry in movement due to the pelvis being aligned differently.

My strength and conditioning sessions were planned, overseen and assisted by an expert trainer who monitored the quality of movement and imbalances as I worked through a set of exercises three to five times per week. Using the rehab and physio exercises as a foundation, the focus in strength and conditioning work was to improve strength for endurance and strength for cycling, swimming and running. I regarded strength and conditioning sessions as essential to overcome the obvious imbalances left to right, attempting to work on patterning and connections across a range of sports-related movement. Throughout the pre-training process, addressing the compensatory issues was a consistent focus.

Importance of strength training:

When an athlete comes to me after trauma I will look for the imbalances in the hips and the torso and use a string of stabilising exercises to strengthen those two areas. Next, I will use unilateral exercises to bring strength in and around the weakened areas and finally use bi-lateral exercises to strengthen the body through plyometric, dynamic and functional movements. Without the strength training the injured party would not recover the body's balance.

How to overcome imbalances left and right or lateral and bilaterally:

After trauma, there will be serious atrophy of the muscles involved and muscles that have a supportive role (synergists) to those involved. These sometimes get neglected during the rehab stages, so when the athlete returns to fitness the synergists are weakened.

The body will naturally adopt a 'new' pathway to cope with loss due to trauma. This should be encouraged because it means all the other muscles and muscle groups can continue to work and keep up their strength. Obviously some muscles will work somewhat harder than others owing to compensatory movement and support.

Athletes generally get back to full strength quicker than non-athletes because their muscles were strong prior to injury, and the compensation wasn't that great or that long.

Tremay Dobson, *elite running trainer, sports therapist and personal trainer*

23 June 2013

I celebrated the benchmark of arriving at a year after the accident in my summer base of the French Alps. A close family friend, Chris, joined me from Australia for the final preparations for the Grand Alps tour. We enjoyed a few acclimatisation rides, and it was great to be back riding long alpine climbs again.

Neuromuscular pathways:

'That breakthrough session is often when the "flow" of movement returns, the emotional connection or "ding" moment happens for the athlete. This greatly enhances the success cycle.'

Tania Cotton, *movement analyst, British chartered physiotherapist*

I felt like I had successfully bridged the void between injury and function, occasionally getting the sense that the flow and rhythm had returned when ascending long climbs. It was a breakthrough session making clear the neuromuscular pathways were working effectively and a well-timed confidence boost before undertaking the week-long cycle from Lake Annecy to the Mediterranean with a group of cyclists.

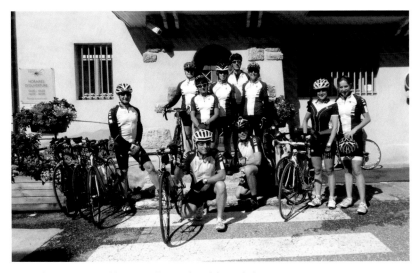

Group departure on Triathlon Europe's 2013 'Aussie' Grand Alps tour

Day 1 – Sunday 30 June 2013

Lake Annecy to Beaufort (92 km)
Climbs: Col des Aravis – 11.5 km, 1486 m elevation
Col des Saises – 14.8 km and 1650 m elevation

After a successful recce ride with the group the day before, a welcome evening dinner and much packing and repacking of bags to locate essential kit, we set off from the hotel in Talloires on Lake Annecy. The group of Australian riders had signed up for their first experience of cycling in the Alps two years ago and had committed to significant preparation for the once-in-a-lifetime ride across the Alps. Significant organisation and effort had gone into getting the trip underway on my side, as the provider, coach and guide as standard on all training weeks in France. Personally and professionally there couldn't have been more elements resting on this week being successful. The pressure was on, and it was an environment I thrived in.

I relished the challenges of the week ahead as I led the group out on the first climb, setting a very easy pace so I could keep the group together and capture images with my camera while I rode. The backdrop of the lake behind the cycling jerseys pedalling around the curves and switchbacks made a vivid sight. I felt back at one with the bike, finding an easy comfort pedalling the rhythm of a light gear up the first demi col leading us away from Lake Annecy.

All three of my team supporting this trip were highly experienced at riding in the mountains and on alpine cols. Having Tania beside me on the first day was indescribably positive and brought recognisable symmetry to my recovery journey one year after the accident.

I felt confident having significantly more support than I would usually need on the road to cover all eventualities. I had prepared myself for the possibility that I might need to make use of the support van during the trip, if my injuries were unable to cope with the consecutive six- to eight-hour cycling days.

It was a great relief to arrive at our quaint hotel after two hour-long climbs, lunch in between and a lovely long descent into the deep valley of Beaufort. Monitoring and assessing each rider's capabilities throughout the day kept me focused on work and helped to start constructing feedback and key points for the subsequent days of the tour.

Once the riders and bikes were attended to, I happily acknowledged that there had been no injury distractions, pain or issues during the 4.5 hours riding on the bike. With comfort breaks, lunch and regrouping at the top of cols, an average day in the mountains covers 80 to 100 kilometres with an average group of riders. My prior assessment in the lead-up to the tour of this level not proving overly demanding on my stage of recovery seemed accurate. I was delighted and on a high; it was so good to be back on track!

The last and most important element of my day was to find time for my usual routine of stretching and mobilising my back and hips. This took just half an hour although I could have easily kept going once I used the foam roller to counter stretch my spine and shoulders. I hope the quality of beds in the hotels we stayed in would be adequate as we rode south; this would be another key aspect of maintaining function for all-day cycling over mountains.

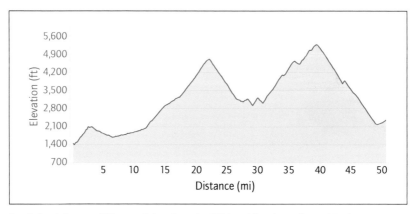

Day 1: Total distance: 85 km, total elevation gain: 2120 m, riding time: 4 hours, 25 minutes

Day 2 – Monday 1 July 2013

Beaufort to Aigueblanche – Bellecombe (85 km)
Climb: Cormet de Roselend – 21 km, 1967 m elevation

After breakfast we set off in two groups to tackle the lengthy but rewarding over 20-kilometre climb of the Cormet de Roseland. I planned to ride with each cyclist and provide some feedback on gearing and climbing techniques in follow-up to observations and discussions from the first day. Such a long climb was perfect for this coaching task. A coffee stop overlooking the barrage Roseland and lunch at the summit provided breaks every two to three hours of cycling.

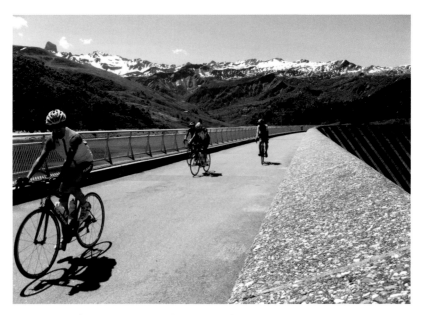

Midway ascent of Cormet de Roselend after morning coffee stop to regroup

Having a relatively novice group was perfect for my stage of recovery as I was able to gain respite to stop and stretch regularly and mobilise my back and body. Riding through relatively low-level pain was manageable on the second day with the regular stops and utilising both standing and sitting climbing techniques on the long ascent.

A technical team time trial along valley roads brought the group into the hotel for the second evening. It had been an extremely hot day on the road, even by Australian standards!

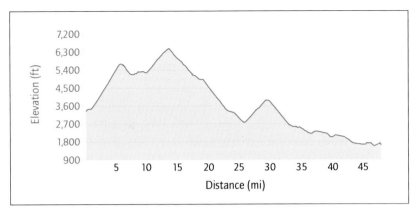

Day 2: Total distance: 78 km, total elevation gain: 1672 m, riding time: 4 hours, 15 minutes

Day 3 – Tuesday 2 July 2013

Aigueblanche – Bellecombe to Oz en Oisans (111 km)
Climbs: Col de la Madeleine – 28 km, 2000 m
Col du Glandon 21.3 km, 1924 m elevation

An uncomfortable bed in the second night hotel set off my back into discomfort from the very start of the day, which didn't improve over the two substantial climbs on our waterproof map profile plan. It was going to be a challenging day leading the group over two huge giants of the Tour de France. Leaning forward to pick up my overnight bag, carrying anything more than the weight of my 7 kg featherweight bike or twisting were options that I had to carefully contemplate to avoid a painful reaction.

With the Tour passing through the same roads in a matter of weeks, our first climb of the day necessitated some off-road variation. The Col de la Madeleine was closed to traffic, and the only way to the summit involved going 'off-piste'. This common summer mountain road scenario challenged even the most well-developed sense of humour; hot sticky tarmac, rising daily temperature, no support van behind us and negotiating narrow trails at the edge of a mountain road in bike shoes with cleats.

Adventure safely accomplished with the group safely carrying their bikes and skirting through fields, it was time to push the pedals to summit in much cooler temperatures at over 1500 metres. An excellent picnic lunch location restored all sense of humour. Well-stocked 'real food', local French produce, salad and fruit replenished energy levels and smiles. Morale-boosting chocolate always wins on difficult days in the mountains, particularly when faced with another big climb before checking into the hotel for the evening!

An excellent long descent off the second col brought us into the village of Oz en Oisans, in the shadow of the famous Alpe D'Huez. I was pleased to have factored in a rest day off the bike, as it would be much needed along with a sports massage!

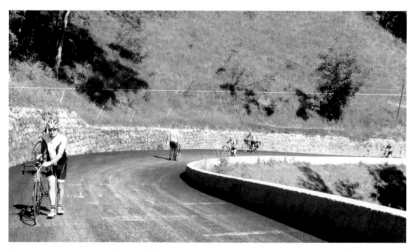

New tarmac for Le Tour de France 2013 provides new dimension to challenge on the climb

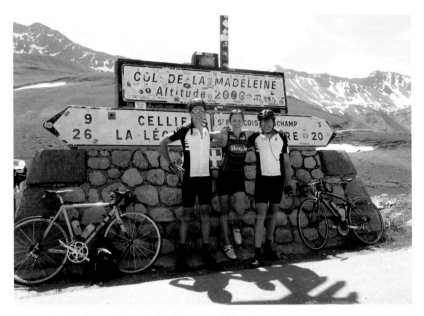

Summit of Col de la Madeleine with leading group of riders

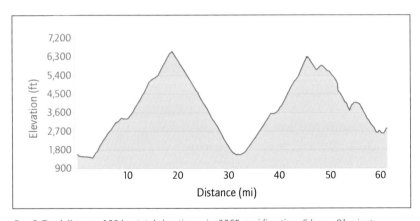

Day 3: Total distance: 100 km, total elevation gain: 3365 m, riding time: 6 hours, 01 minute

Day 4 – Wednesday 3 July 2013

Oz en Oisans – One-day stay
Climb: Alpe D'Huez – 13.2 km, 1860 m

With an unhappy body, I took a break from the bike for 24 hours. It made sense to draw upon the experience of numerous rehab hours and apply the enhanced repair benefits to have me back on the bike the following day. Adding to the pain accumulation at this early stage would put me in serious doubt of completing the Grand Alps tour with so many more mountains left to lead the group over.

With the riders keen to take on L'Alpe D'Huez and our itinerary planned for the one-day stay at a beautifully equipped chalet, I had the luxury of regularly stretching, a sports massage and manipulating the painful areas in my back and pelvis with heat therapy morning, noon and night. My van driver and support riders supported the group to ascend L'Alpe D'Huez with lunch at the summit and exploration time.

A rainy day and wet roads made it an easy decision for me not to take any unnecessary risks to cycle up a mountain I had ridden and descended numerous times.

It was a shame as I had highly recommended this climb to the group at the early planning stages two years ago. We had adapted the classic Route des Grandes Alpes itinerary to accommodate a day at the foot of the mountain in order for them to ride it. So they enjoyed testing their newly developed climbing and descending skills on the 21 hairpin switchbacks of the iconic climb seen many times in the TV coverage of the Tour in Australia, despite the summer rain!

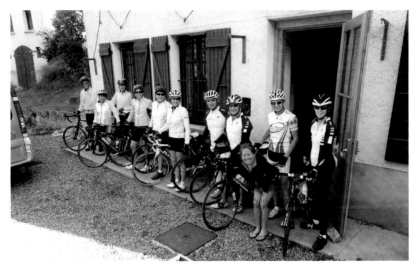

Aussie group depart from Oz, after conquering L'Alpe D'Huez

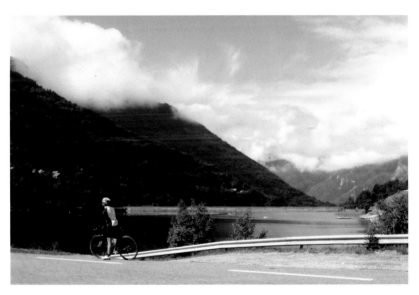

Regular breaks every two hours to stretch out injury sites and admire the views

Day 5 – Thursday 4 July 2013

Oz en Oisans to Briancon – 70 km
Climb: Col du Lautaret – 25 km, 2058 m

Having spent two nights sleeping on a decent mattress and bed helped alleviate some of the back issues. Loading bags and moving or carrying luggage compounded some of the issues. It was, however, good to be back on the bike. My fatigue levels had subsided with the benefit of a rest day from cycling. The first climb encouraged the group to spread out and ride at their own pace, and a picnic lunch waited at the top of the climb. Fatigue levels were noticeable in many of the group on the second, shorter climb after lunch.

A rest day in the lovely town of Briancon was planned the following day for everyone, and sports massages were pre-booked. I needed to use pain medication later in the evening to sleep.

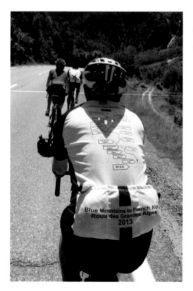

Aidan's, the ride guide, col map-backed jersey to assist navigation

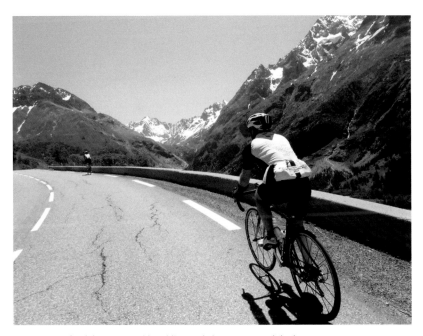

Final ascent of Col du Lautaret, riders riding at their own pace and rhythm

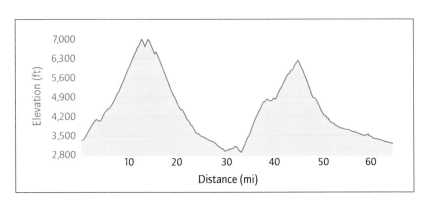

Day 5: Total distance: 67 km, total elevation gain: 2202 m, riding time: 3 hours, 35 minutes

Day 6 – Friday 5 July 2013

Rest day – Briancon

This was the dedicated rest day of the trip and marked our halfway point on the route. The riders spent the day off their bikes, exploring the contrasting medieval and modern town of Briancon. I had arranged a massage therapist to provide sports massages. The bikes were given a check over and clean. It was important to have reliable, well-maintained equipment on the climbs and the descents, particularly.

I enjoyed my usual morning routine of stretching, mobilising and activating glutes, balance, posture and core, with full knowledge I did not have to subject myself to any pressure or pain sitting on a bike saddle for four to six hours. This recovery ritual was repeated again in the evening, and some walking around acting as a tour guide up and down the steep hill to lunch in the beautiful medieval part of town proved a good way to stretch out the legs. The hotel bed was excellent, and it was helpful to have a full two nights' rest before taking on the second half of the tour to the Mediterranean.

Mountain mindset:

My advice to anyone riding in the alps, first-timer or experienced rider, is that it is far better to adopt a can-do approach of 'ride as you find it'.

Having this perspective will ensure you ride at your own pace and find a rhythm that suits you and your level of fitness or how strong you are feeling on the day.

This is particularly relevant if you are riding from point to point on a Grand Alps tour where you have huge variations in terrain and climbs for four to eight hours a day.

Without preconceived ideas about the level of difficulty or what is ahead, you can then focus the most important muscle, the mind, on the job of pedalling and maintaining sustainable effort and fuelling or hydration at regular intervals.

If you are having a bad day, it is amazing how a five-minute rest on the side of a mountain road admiring the views will provide you with the perspective and strength to get you through the rough patch and back on the road to the summit.

Day 7 – Saturday 6 July 2013

Briancon to Barcelonnette (104 km)
Climbs: Col d'Izoard – 20 km, 2361 m
Col de Vars – 19 km, 2128 m

It was a challenging day on the road with the group split into two and allocating support riders without the van. The climbs were scenic and the group rode well after a day off. We arrived late to the hotel as a result of a van issue just before the weather closed in. The evening meal and accommodation was excellent to compensate. Once again I could just about manage the constant pain from my lower back and right side of my pelvis from another day in the saddle.

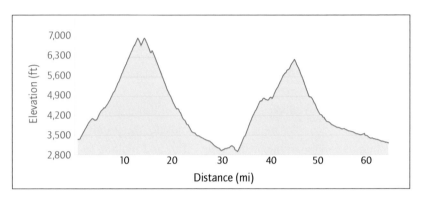

Day 7: Total distance: 104 km, total elevation gain: 2413 m, riding time: 5 hours, 40 minutes

Day 8 – Sunday 7 July 2013

Barcelonette to Roure – 90 km
Climbs: Col de la Cayolle – 29 km, 2326 m
Col de la Couillole – 29 km, 1678 m

Two beautiful climbs on quieter roads, both of reasonable gradient with the first of them a giant over 2000 metres at the summit. I had been looking forward to this day on the route! My legs and strength had returned, and I enjoyed leading from the front, encouraging Chris to push new limits on a mutually favourite col we had both ridden before.

The group were increasingly becoming independent and enjoying the ease of navigating the Route des Grandes Alpes from the familiar signs on the roads, each other's jerseys and waterproof pocket maps I had prepared for them. It was efficient and effective for me to be able to start at the back of the group slowly to warm up, riding with each in turn briefly to check with how they were progressing and pedalling before making my way through to the front of the group with short efforts. It was an extended interval session, giving me regular recovery to take photos of riders and mountain views to capture the tour in pictures. All the practice I had doing things single-handedly was put to good use!

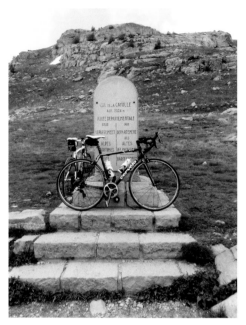

My favourite 'big chain ring challenge' col. The Col de la Cayolle's moderate average gradient for 20 kilometres, makes it ideal for developing muscular strength and endurance for over an hour.

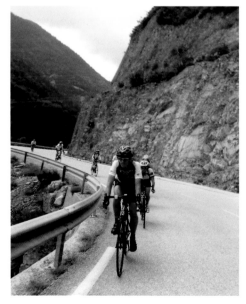

Group ascending the climb of two halves, the Col de la Couillole

It was rewarding to see the riders implementing the climbing and descending advice and improving immeasurably in confidence and technical abilities. This particular route was one I liked to use each year with a specific brief to each rider to put particular skills into practice over sustained climbs and lengthy but quite safe descents.

Our hotel tucked away at the top of a cheeky 5-kilometre climb from the valley floor was well worth the effort, although some encouragement was needed to make this final haul after an eight-hour ride day. This was a little detail I would only disclose at lunchtime, after we had banked one of the biggest cols in the Alps. The hotel is literally a highlight, in every possible sense!

My morning and evening stretching, strengthening and mobilising rituals were working well, and my lower back responded well to a night in a comfortable bed.

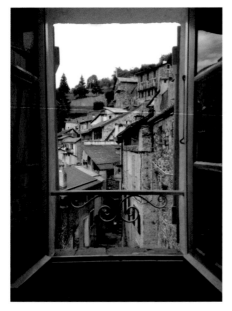

Waking up to beautiful views in Ruore, before the penultimate day cycling to the Mediterranean

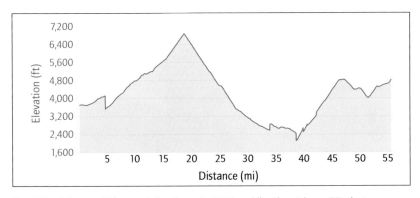

Day 8: Total distance: 90 km, total elevation gain: 2432 m, riding time: 5 hours, 15 minutes

Day 9 – Monday 8 July 2013

Ruore to Sospel – 90 km
Climb: Col Saint-Martin – 16.5 km, 1500 m
Col de Turini – 15 km, 1607 m

After a celebratory evening and excellent stay in a unique, boutique hotel, we descended confidently as a group on narrow, twisty roads to the valley floor. All along the road beside the river were signs tempting us to the Mediterranean via Nice; however, our route took us over two smaller cols.

I was delighted to be on the bike with the end in sight, optimistic that I would manage to ride the trip successfully with the last huge day behind us. It felt like a major accomplishment to have pushed through the challenges to ascend just three more baby cols to finish on the beach in a day's time!

However, the mountains had one more little test for us.

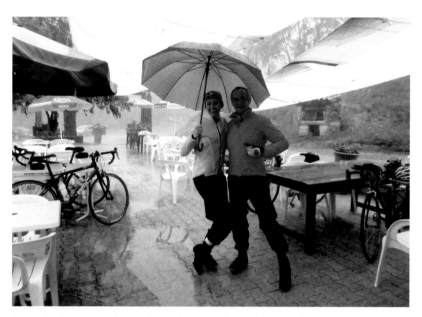

Prepare for all seasons and eventualities when cycling in the high mountains.

Our penultimate day involved cycling close to the Italian border and enjoying different scenery on the two relatively smaller climbs. The weather had become a lot warmer as we ventured south during the week, and we experienced a heavy thunderstorm on the final big col of the week. We sought shelter to regroup while the thunder and lightning descended on the mountaintop to minimise the risk of descending on flooded roads off a high col. Our final stay was in a hilltop hotel in Sospel.

We had a celebratory final evening focused on all of the individual achievements of the group on their first epic cycling trip. They had managed a huge challenge, and all of their preparation for nearly two years had paid off. I was very proud of them.

Reflecting on how far I had come to be back on track personally and professionally and able to lead the tour successfully was an emotional experience. It had been a six-month goal for me to prepare on every level, starting from a much lower base than my clients. I had prescribed their training to complete in the Blue Mountains, west of Sydney, and had barely been able to follow the training plan I had created for them at times during the lead-up to this tour.

When we had set off from Lake Annecy a week earlier, I had fully intended to split my time on the bike and in the van if my recovering injuries dictated. It was amazing to consider that the last day would be the culmination of all personal journeys to complete the Grand Alps tour, and I had been back on the bike almost every day.

Day 10 – Tuesday 9 July 2013

Sospel to Menton – 20 km
Climbs: Col de Castillon – 7 km, 706 m

After some photos and co-ordinating the group's departure kit for our final day, we cycled over the final small col straight out of the hotel. As we cycled the final few kilometres through the town of Menton, the smell of the sea and Mediterranean drew us towards our beach destination.

It was both a relief and a highlight to finish the tour, with the group accomplishing a once-in-a-lifetime achievement by bike. My support team had been brilliant in working together to facilitate all the physical aspects that I would usually do. The sea, sand and sun provided a nice swim, and after lunch it was time to pack up the bikes and get everyone to the airport or hotel in Nice.

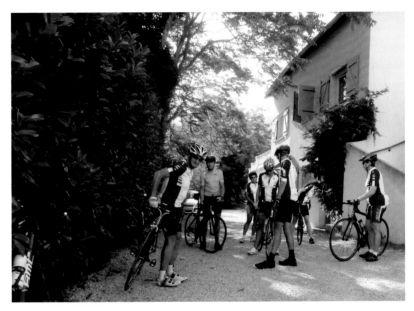

Final day departure, preparing for hot conditions

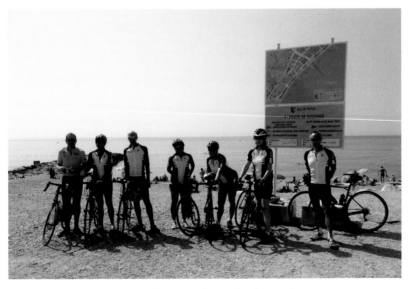

The Mediterranean final destination of the Route des Grandes Alpes 2013

I made the flight back to London from Nice very happy for the group, thankful for my support crew and unable to believe the journey had ended and the scale of what I had managed to do, just a year on from sustaining the injuries. It was hard to believe that from no mobility or independence I was now firmly at the other end of the scale.

I looked forward to a few very easy weeks off the bike to allow all the aches and soreness to settle down. I knew that my body needed time to absorb the punishing days, and I was grateful for it being able to rise to the challenges every day. It had been an amazing few weeks on many levels. Scaling the beautiful climbs in the Alps, professionally back leading my training weeks and completing all of the days on the bike over the mountains was worth celebrating.

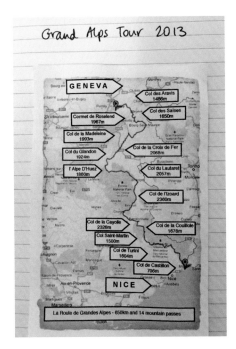

The Grand Alps Tour 2013 was a huge turning point in my recovery, reinforcing belief and providing much needed boost in motivation to keep going despite significant financial pressure to consider practical, less physical options for work and my career path.

Grand Alps Tour 2013

Going further?

Following severe injures sustained at high speed when racing or training, it is possible to discover new performance potential that has been lost or has not yet been uncovered. Accident and injury can provide an opportunity to re-establish better form when combined with sufficiently planned time to recover and rebuild. You can improve your physical capacity by learning and integrating more efficient movement patterns into your training and performance that can give you greater and more sustainable performance gains long term. Form-focused training highlights movement inefficiencies and, through progressive functional training, empowers athletes to develop and optimise their performance potential.

Tania Cotton, *movement analyst, British chartered physiotherapist*

'Acknowledging just how adaptable the body is, if the mind is willing, is the most powerful step you can take to success.'

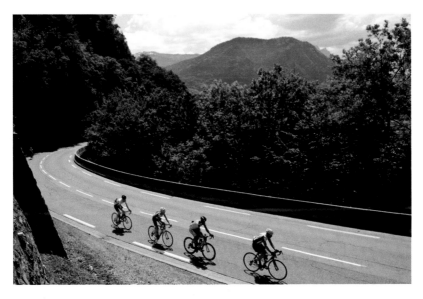

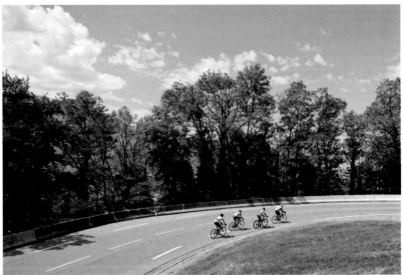

Group riding to ascend Col de Joux-Plane, French Alps Triathlon training week 2012

CHAPTER 9:
BACK ON TRACK

Biggest achievement: Getting back on the start line of a 10K running race

Elevation gain: 0 m
Distance: 10 km

July 2013

Returning from the French Alps was like coming down from a huge post-Ironman® high. Faced with the reality of achieving an amazing physical feat of recovery yet still struggling to regain the thriving coaching business I once had was difficult to manage and compounded the situation.

Analysing my options highlighted that the capability and desire was there to succeed; however, no matter how great this was, I had to be realistic and work out how long I could offset my significant loss of income and increased outgoings the past year. I spent many weeks feeling low with little energy to invest in anything but returning to the routine of work. I was physically exhausted and in the middle of a heightened adaptation process similar to the culmination of a six-month journey to an Ironman® finish line. This allowed me to give myself some slack. Rest was the answer.

My training sessions changed to assist recovery and reduce some of the injury pain in the weeks after the cycle tour. I was not keen to get back on a bike for a few weeks until my pelvis stopped hurting. I focused on completing a water-based session each day in the form of a short swim or aqua run session, my daily strength work and the occasional easy spin on the bike once or twice a week as a form of commuting somewhere to coach or pick up anything I needed from the shops.

I opted for a change and took the mountain bike out on the trails for short rides, which provided a welcome change in position and terrain. It was a way of checking in with the injury site pain and gauging any improvement. After a few weeks I started to reintroduce light runs, starting from the 20-minute easy jog duration from the rehab program. I appreciated the time and space to seek solutions to problems while running. When badly injured this was a time that I didn't have available to me, and gaining it back was of huge benefit in processing ideas and options to identify how I was going to keep myself going financially.

Over the late summer I decided to invest in a cheap, recycled vintage bike with panniers to carry bags and equipment. It meant I could consider selling my much-loved sports car to provide some cash flow for a few months and pay my bills.

Things were getting tough. I couldn't physically work any more hours, already stretched coaching evenings, working Sundays twice a month and my daily work with athlete plans, admin or coaching. Although the business was gradually improving and getting back to approximately 50% of pre-accident levels of income, it was looking like it would not be sustainable much beyond a few more months to the end of the year. I delayed putting my car up for sale until the New Year; I couldn't bear to part with it in this way. I had purchased it with the combined funds of a final company bonus before I left my job as a consultant to set up my business and saved prize money earnings. Instead I went with a short-term solution in having a 'fire sale', getting rid of kit and gear I no longer needed for racing and training. I decided minimalistic and some extra cash was a positive and necessary outcome of this stage in recovery. It provided a much needed lift!

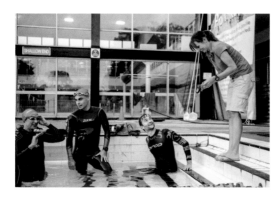

Providing individual coaching feedback to squad swimmers

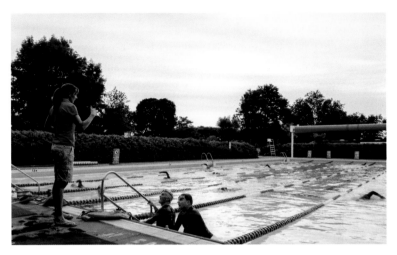

Coaching SwimSmooth squad, South West London

August 2013

I had a few celebrations around the time of my birthday, bringing all of my friends together who had helped me through the time of the accident and critical recovery months to thank them personally. Taking the time to acknowledge the vast group of people who had been such positive support helped to focus on how far I had come with the collective help. It was also a welcome distraction to another imminent operation to remove the clavicle plate from my shoulder at the end of the summer.

More practically on a daily basis, the plate in my shoulder was uncomfortable when resting and protruded with pain at either end of the clavicle if I forgot and rolled onto the right shoulder. Carrying a bag or wearing a seatbelt over the right shoulder were both problematic. I was aware that if I had another fall from my bike while cycling and landed on that shoulder, there would be complications if I broke anything with the plate attached to the clavicle. A small risk, I hoped, and I didn't consider it when descending any high mountains!

The plate restricted my range of movement in my right arm when swimming, and I had modified my arm recovery accordingly. Optimal body rotation to both sides was key to not regularly causing impingement when I swam my sets. If I swam with my hips or shoulders relatively flat in the water, usually on my longer swims, then it would start to become a problem. Additionally swimming with masters involved some medley strokes, and it was very difficult performing butterfly strokes again with the plate in situ. My sleeping position had been adapted, as it was no longer possible to sleep on my right side. Out running, my shoulder would ache from the jarring or plate, or both. A walk would soon resolve the pain, and I could jog lightly again. At a routine follow-up appointment with my consultant surgeon, he recommended it should be removed after a year as it had served its purpose in helping the clavicle to mend successfully.

In the weeks leading up to the operation I made the necessary provisions to scale down work commitments and arrange coaching cover for the evening sessions. It certainly didn't help my anxiety about finances, knowing I had to reduce earnings for a week or two post-surgery. My motivation levels to swim were particularly low, in the knowledge my current hard-earned swimming fitness and re-established technique would be set back significantly in the eight-week recovery period post operation. At least I knew what I had to do to rehab afterwards! It would be a much more straightforward process with a shorter recovery timescale compared to reconstructing the shoulder on the first operation. I dusted off my sling in preparation for reuniting it with my right arm for a few weeks.

The operation was a day procedure, and I was home in the evening. Inspecting the surgery wound in the follow-up appointment a week later revealed it was quite untidy. I wondered if a student doctor had performed the less complicated operation to remove the clavicle plate, as the finishing scar lacked the neat finish of the first surgeon's work.

Along the surgical wound, my skin was gathered unevenly at one end, a wide diagonal red line had appeared across the front of my shoulder from under the wound to my neckline and a significant amount of soft tissue seemed distributed lumpily above the scar. The whole area was much more sensitive than I expected, and the nerve endings down my arm were numb and tingly. It felt as though the plate had been removed with difficulty, as the area surrounding it was quite disturbed. I hoped over time the body would work its magic on repairing this invasion on the shoulder for a second time.

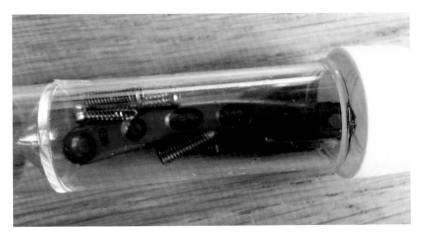

Surgical plate 120 x 15 x 5 mm to repair clavicle and 20 mm screws

The week after surgery involved the usual challenges of trying to manage single-handedly. Painstakingly trying to shower without getting the shoulder dressing wet and care for long hair necessitated a trip to the hairdressers for a shampoo and blow dry. It would be a number of weeks before I could lift my right arm above my shoulder to perform this simple task. Preparing meals with one arm and operating with a single hand for work reminded me of all the coping strategies I had developed last summer. Except this time I was better able to function or move easily and had prepared in advance.

Post-operation I was unexpectedly very tired for more than the first few days, reintroducing my afternoon nap regime where possible. I was given pain medication to take for a week after the operation but opted to not use tramadol and stuck with ibuprofen and paracetemol instead. Work was minimised in the weeks afterwards as my fatigue levels were not subsiding, due to evening coaching and early morning weekend workshops. Although I was keen to re-establish my training routine and get back in the water swimming, at every opportunity I sought more sleep!

Post surgery:

Returning to a full training load after surgery will obviously depend on the particular surgery and the effects of the surgery on the individual, both physically and mentally. In my own case I regarded both instances of surgery as merely an inconvenience to the training regime. I certainly didn't feel that it would impact on me in the long term and indeed may have provided me with an opportunity to break the routine and perhaps avoid any 'staleness'.

By considering the surgery as simply a temporary incursion into my training I did not allow it to have any negative impact on my mental state. When considering the actual physical training regime, an individual's mental state will determine how the training is undertaken.

On the two occasions I have made a return to training, after two weeks and on the second time after six weeks, my aim was to complete the entire session working as hard as possible. My theory was that this method would allow me to get back to full fitness as quickly as possible, but this may not suit everyone!

An alternative approach would be to gradually work up to full capacity over an extended period of time; it's physically easier and the end result may well be the same. It depends on the individual

It is very much about the individual knowing him- or herself and how they train. This is going to impact on how they recover.

Chris Fidler, *British record long course, British record short course x2, European record short course x2*

Rehabilitating back into training:

>> Meet with your coach, doctor, physio and strength coach so that everybody is on the same page with your rehabilitation.

>> Listen to your body. Avoid pushing through pain in movement or strengthening work. With surgery you have to rest and take time off training; another few days off is a small sacrifice in the big picture if something flares up.

>> Utilise this time wisely to come back stronger than before. Turn a negative into a positive by taking the time to turn a physical weakness into a strength.

Coping strategies:

>> Make small goals so things don't seem too far away. Instead of just having the end goal a race in a year's time, focus on something in 6 months time, and then 7 months, etc., so you can have something to look forward to along the way.

>> Appreicate that a career can last 10 years, and every now and then you're bound to have ups and downs. Many greats have had their fair share of setbacks, but what separates them from the rest is how they respond to hardships.

>> Remove yourself from the sport. If it bothers you hearing about results from other athletes, then concentrate on getting your rehab done and focus on what YOU can do.

Ryan Gregson, *Olympic 1500-metre runner and Australian record holder*

Managing recovery and rehabilitation:

>> After undergoing surgery for an injury your body is extremely weak, so it's important to be patient with the road back to recovery. Listen to your physio and sports doctor before trying to jump back into a full training regime. The chance of causing another injury is very likely. Rest is the first critical sage of recovery.

>> Work out a strict rehab programme that concentrates on bringing your body back to full strength. This may take weeks or months, but you can't advance back to your full training load until your body can handle the stress.

>> Before starting back to training make sure your coach and physio agree on what you can handle. They must agree on where you are in regards to training load so if anything pops up, it can be addressed immediately and correctly.

Strategies to cope with setbacks as you return to competitive form:

» The biggest part about setbacks or delays in your usual training is mentally accepting what race or training you had to miss out on or sacrifice due to the injury. If you dwell on the immediate future, the thought of returning to training can seem daunting. Focus first on getting yourself right the smartest and fastest way possible.

» Create a calendar that outlines each big step coming up in regards to returning to training. Break it down into small goals so you can focus on what you can do at the present time rather than getting overwhelmed about how far away full recovery seems.

» Use the little extra downtime you have from training to take notes and write down how you could become even stronger from this injury. You now have a chance to perfect any little faults in your training or gym programme, so work out how you can become better, faster and stronger from the injury by altering your rehab programme.

Genevieve LaCaze, *Australian distance athlete (3000-metre steeplechase), 2012 Olympian, 2014 5th place at the Glasgow Commonwealth Games*

September 2013

Working under the supervision of the hospital physiotherapist, my arm was confined to a sling for two weeks with gradual introduction of movement through the hand and elbow. As the weeks went by I resumed the progression of reintroducing more range of movement through to shoulder height and then finally after six weeks above my shoulder. It was great to be back swimming every morning with Chris, Geoff and Paul. I was always greatly inspired by their longevity in the sport of swimming and achievements as British and European record holders. Their encouragement and dedication echoed my training mindset to see the positives and to keep swimming! The routine each morning with a group was highly motivating and demanded commitment, at any stage of the recovery process. Excuses were unnecessary once the session got underway.

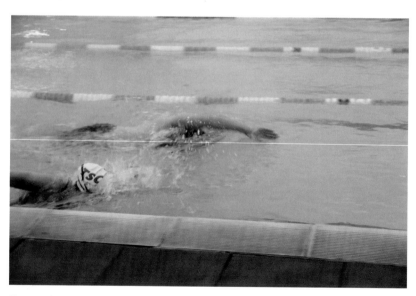

The commitment to train with a similar ability group of athletes enhances motivation to overcome setbacks post surgery or injury.

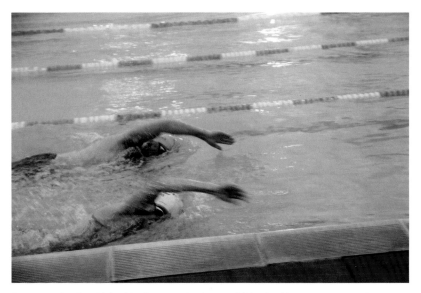

Pace sets swimming side by side, demonstrating improved right shoulder range post second surgery

The exercises I worked through each day also helped mobilise my upper back which noticeably became stiff with lack of movement. Although they helped the process of loosening tight and sore muscles around the shoulder, I needed to physically manipulate the area with massage particularly to check in on the extent of numbness down the arm and around the injury site and scar. Once I was able to, I was back in the water, walking, running and completing light pre-training swim sessions without any arm recovery. It felt great to be mobilising my legs, back and body while my shoulder mended, supported by the water.

The wound continued to look puffy and inflamed for eight weeks afterwards. I was away in France running swim workshops for a few days and started to feel unwell. The injury site had been unexpectedly irritated throughout my trip away, more noticeably so due to carrying bags and equipment around. On the flight back to London it felt like something was inside the scar and trying to get out.

Unsurprisingly when I inspected it upon arriving home late at night, it looked infected and swollen. A retained stitch proved to be the culprit, and it was a great relief to remove it myself with a scalpel and tweezers once the wound erupted at one end. I managed to get an emergency appointment with the GP after visiting the pharmacy for a dressing for the weeping wound. An inspection of the issue and course of antibiotics prescribed by the GP was reassuring to check my self-surgery.

Another visit back to the hospital was made in order to check that nothing else was left behind in the wound, allowing the recovery process to run its course. The antibiotics, however, took their toll on my appetite, metabolism and energy in the weeks afterwards, and I made some modifications to my daily nutrition to support this. I was getting a bit tired of all the running around for medical appointments while trying to focus most of my available energy and time supporting myself with consistent work.

An unexpected challenge after my second operation was not a physical one, which made a change. The new challenge was managing expectations of other people around me, who were keen for me to train with them or take on more than I felt comfortable doing. I discovered that my perception of unnecessary risk was far more conservative in order to not have an impact on my daily pain management and ultimately my livelihood. It had taken 18 months, many hours of physiotherapy, rehab exercises, being patient and immeasurable worry about whether my business would survive such a catastrophic setback, without adding anything remotely similar into the equation!

I became more accustomed to declining activities and opportunities to train with others I didn't know or taking on activities I thought weren't worth provoking my injuries over. It was a balancing act guided by intuition. My surgeon had cautioned that I needed to be careful not to fall on my shoulder in 8 to 12 weeks post surgery as the clavicle would be fragile until it compensated for the screw holes where the plate had been attached. So declining invitations to go mountain biking off road or running up and down hills and trails was not difficult. I had enough challenges in injury management after fairly conservative training sessions, compared to my previous abilities to run for two to three hours at altitude or cycle 100 miles over mountains in Ironman® training. Constantly reminding myself of where I was now, rather than expecting to meet other people's expectations of what I used to be able to easily do, was a raw process of adjustment.

It took some getting used to having my new outlook on outdoor sport, particularly when dealing with pressure to do activities I would have undertaken without a second thought pre-accident and recovery. My horizons had changed, and unless activities directly related to my coaching work or personal rehabilitation, I simply didn't want to risk causing any form of pain escalation, further medical complications or disruption from my consistent daily investment in strength and conditioning.

All the work I had done had progressed me from immobile to functional. I couldn't have been happier about where I had recovered to and was not going to deviate from this road to satisfy anyone else's perception of what was ok for me! I also felt I wasn't missing out on anything, having spent years racing at international level and taken risks in training and performance terms when needed to achieve the best I was capable of.

Having the financial pressure hanging over me on a weekly basis greatly influenced this mindset, too. I still had to come up with a solution to the financial problems I was facing or implement more drastic measures such as moving out of my home and seeking a normal 9-5 day job. I could not afford another setback, however minor.

Resist going 'off piste' until you are ready to.

1. Go beyond listening to your body; know it inside and out. Seek feedback from areas that are mending and recovering through functional exercises and form focus in training.

2. Have a 'road map' for your recovery, rehabilitation and pre-training back to full training or competition. There will be more than one route, however!

3. Use your regular sessions to consistently see progression towards where you want to be.

4. Recognise that peers and training friends are likely operating at a higher physical level.

5. Resist pressure to train as others are or to undertake activities that you sense might be too much of a 'stretch' at any stage of your recovery process.

6. Avoid justifying a 'no' to any training opportunities that may set you back. It is a visual assumption that you appear 'fixed' and recovered from your injuries. Many more layers make up recovery, however!

7. Use your own custom equipment, particularly if you have adapted your bike setup. Borrowed equipment often causes reaction from injuries due to significant positional changes from what your injuries have adapted to.

8. Develop independence to get on with your plan; 'stealth' training is an effective strategy.

9. Have confidence that you alone know what is best for you and your capabilities at the time.

10. Choose your experts and advisors carefully based on experience and relevance to your situation or sport.

Post-surgery advice and recommendations:

In June 2013 I was as high as a kite from just having won the biggest race of my career, the 46-kilometre Manhattan Island Marathon Swim. I had trained brilliantly for the event, and everything went according to plan. I felt on top of the world.

Just six weeks later, however, I somehow suffered a disc prolapse in L4/5 of my lower back which stopped me walking properly for nearly six months due to extreme sciatic pain in my right leg. I still don't know how I did it. Even basic interactions on the floor playing with my kids were impossible. It's fair to say I became quite depressed about this whole situation as I'd set myself some lofty goals after winning the race. None of the physiotherapy and Pilates interventions seemed to be working despite everyone's best efforts to assist me.

It was a very rough period for me and one in which I couldn't see light at the end of 'tunnel' until the prospect of neurosurgery in the form of a micro-disectomy with one of the world's leading surgeons in this field (Dr. Stephen Lewis) fortunately presented itself. Many asked *'Aren't you scared of back surgery – you might never walk again!'* but I knew simply that this was very much my last resort and the only thing that would get me back to full health. As soon as I awoke from surgery I knew the problem had been fixed. It was like a light switch had been flicked, and I could then start the process of rehab, both physically and psychologically.

Once I knew the 'road block' had been cleared I could look positively forward at how to rehab myself back to full training. I felt I had the ultimate training plan from my win in Manhattan and that I'd just have to be patient and start slowly working my way back into it. Sure enough, I have. It's precisely 12 months ago since I had the surgery, and I am swimming better now than I have ever done in my life, setting a lifetime best for a 5-kilometre open water event on the anniversary of going under the knife.

I strongly believe that it was the positivity of knowing I was fixed with the necessity for extreme patience that got me back on the road to full health, and I couldn't feel any better now. I accepted the setback and embraced the challenge of the rehabilitation and have come out the other side all the better for it!

Paul Newsome, *Owner, SwimSmooth 2013 Manhattan Island Marathon Swim champion*

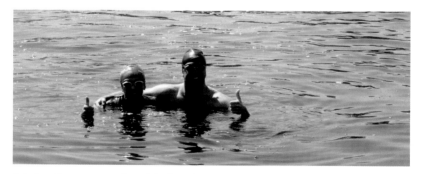

SwimSmooth open water swim training in Perth, Australia

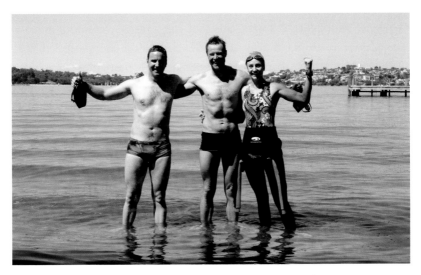

Set a realistic approach and celebrate any increment of progress in every session.

December 2013

Transitioning back to multisport training at an easy level over the winter months helped overcome the lack of motivation I had experienced after the build-up to the summer Alps tour.

Reviewing and improving the gradated rehabilitation plan took this to another level, and I started to put together a new road map for the year ahead. Having a major goal on the horizon helped to focus my rehabilitation back onto the bike in the year after the accident, and the road map provided a flexible way of working with non-linear progress. The key components were a weekly training schedule that was made up of strength and conditioning, yoga, swimming and some running and cycling. I was keen to see if I could toe a start line of a running event, cycling event and swimming event as separate sports before considering a full comeback to a triathlon.

Focusing training at different times of the year or season, similar to 'periodisation' in traditional coaching terms for endurance athletes, seemed an obvious solution for managing multisport training without having to do everything at once, all year round. It was a key component of coaching athletes, and I enjoyed creating bespoke annual plans around races, taking into account their performance profiles.

Employing this approach to my pre-training and ongoing rehabilitation to see whether I could progress sufficiently without lasting issues to injuries into to competitive sport would be motivating to see what it would yield. I had another warm weather break in Australia over Christmas and returned feeling less pain from the injuries as last time, and with a plan!

March 2014

For three months I made good progress with swimming, running and strength focus. My aim was to complete a local 5-kilometre park run by Easter, and I increased my run training to three sessions of 40 to 70 minutes per week from short 20-minute sessions. It was great to be running at a steady, sustainable pace again; one of the best outcomes was having time to find solutions to problems. It was time well spent, gaining a creativity and energy boost at the same time.

I had settled into an early-morning routine of swimming every day, with an accomplished group of national and European record-winning masters swimmers at my local health gym and club. Within three months of consistent training I had regained my sustainable speed and endurance of previous levels. I was logging up to 20 kilometres a week in training, with a slightly modified technique. It was working well, and the speed returned quite quickly after a few weeks working strongly similar levels pre-surgery.

Having a video analysis on my stroke six months into the recovery process was fundamental in assessing where asymmetry presented itself due to the injuries. Making modifications to body rotation range as my core strength improved and relaxing the arm recovery to alleviate the shoulder operation and plate were instrumental in achieving previous form and speeds in training. I planned a summer race when the open water opportunities presented themselves to gain a benchmark under race conditions.

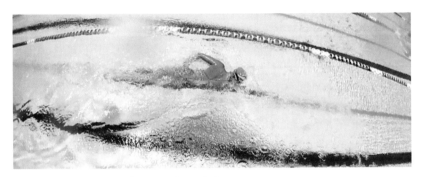

SwimSmooth video analysis of body rotation and alignment

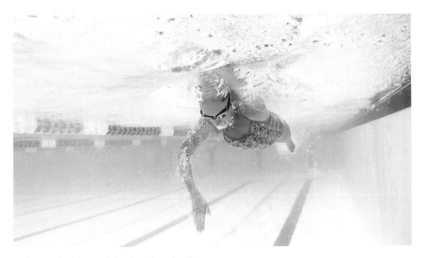

SwimSmooth video analysis of catch and pull

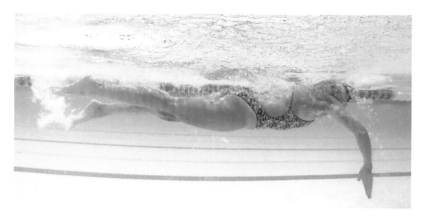

SwimSmooth video analysis of body and leg position

One of the highlights of my winter swim training was having Paul Newsome, owner of SwimSmooth in Australia and triathlon legend Dave Scott join us one morning to swim. They were both in town for the triathlon show, and it was great to meet Dave and catch up with Paul. This was a breakthrough swim session, pushing the boundaries of what pain had limited me to before in training and feeling strong throughout.

My injuries were a little creaky afterwards, and more attention to stretching out in the evening helped develop a less painful range for the following day. Paul and Dave joined me again to train with the masters session at Hampton pool, causing quite a stir at the early morning session in the outdoor pool at Hampton!

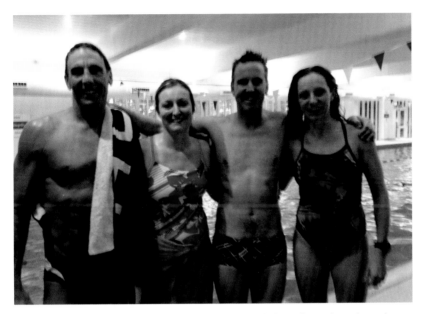

Dave Scott, Annie Oberlin Harris, Paul Newsome and Fiona Ford after early morning swim session

My strength and conditioning workouts were tailored from the range of exercises I had been prescribed, given, implemented and developed progression with. Creating a set of exercises in a wall display reminded me every day to complete a sequence of mobilisation and stabilisation movements using body weight. Repetition over many months had fine-tuned and developed a number of exercises into a session I could do anywhere in 30 minutes.

Most days would start with this before a swim, or I would use the session in the evenings to gently unwind and re-establish symmetry and flexibility in posture and balance. I became addicted to the 'click' to release areas of my spine. One morning in late March I woke up and suddenly realised I no longer had significant back pain from the left side around my sacrum. This was a revelation, nearly two years after the injuries!

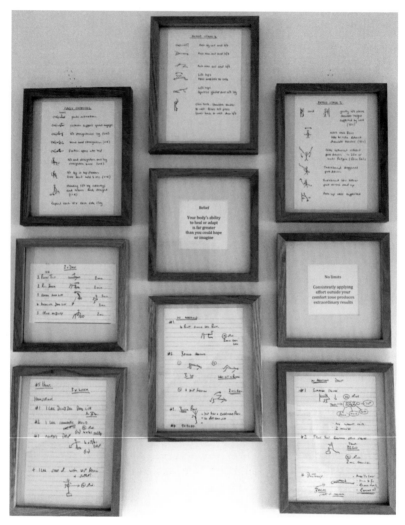

A visual reminder of movement and mobility exercises enhances your commitment to movement rituals every day and provides assessment opportunities to inform your training on any given day.

It had taken over a year after the accident to rebuild my body, and as a result strength and conditioning sessions were now a key part of my new training week. My focus was now on securing a livelihood again.

I had put off the sale of my beloved sports car for a few more months and finally sold it to help solve the financial problems I was having in the short term. I hoped I might buy a replacement if and when the insurance claim against the driver who caused my injuries ever came to fruition.

Putting together the accident and injury claim with my solicitor was a necessary element that suddenly took over all of my available spare time. The process induced a roller coaster of worry, doubts and confidence that it would all work out in the end. There was no definitive timescale for settlement, and it rumbled on in the background of everything else that defined my progress.

My shoulder had healed, with a little disfigurement from a messy surgery wound. As I progressed my running very gradually over the spring months I would occasionally have deep, aching bone pain from the clavicle when running. It would be sufficient enough to have to stop and walk briefly to cease jarring the injury. I looked for particular designs of running tops and bra straps that helped to alleviate the pressure across the collarbone. This was one of the side effects of gaining some weight! My upper right arm remained slightly numb and tingly to touch in places with some referred nerve pain into the collarbone.

With a shift in focus from bike to run over the winter months, I completed three local 5-kilometre timed parkruns.

Fiona FORD (6 parkruns) Most Recent Runs					
Event	Run Date	Gender Pos	Overall Pos	Time	Age Grade
Bushy parkrun	06/09/2014	2	102	20:44	75.88%
Bushy parkrun	08/03/2014	5	108	20:37	75.75%
Bushy parkrun	01/02/2014	5	81	21:16	73.43%
Bushy parkrun	10/12/2011	7	88	19:27	79.09%
Bushy parkrun	01/01/2011	1	30	19:35	78.30%
Bushy parkrun	31/01/2009	1	47	19:44	76.77%

Progress on return to 5-kilometre timed parkrun in 2014

Wednesday 18 June 2014

I put my consistent swim training to the test in July with a very pleasing 22:20 1500-metre open water wetsuit swim. This was only a minute or two off my previous Olympic distance race speed. It was a very nice surprise to figure amongst the podium placings!

I was delighted with the whole experience, being back on a start line in a competitive mindset to see what I could produce on the day. More importantly, only in the lead-up to the event did I think about getting jostled and the impact on my injuries during or after the race. Once I was off and racing, I was focused purely on performance, tactics and how my effort was being maintained on the two-lap swim. A great result, and first stage of the road back to competition. By returning to multisport through a single-sport focus, the areas of training, recovery and mindset could be optimally managed. The next focus would be a running event later in the Autumn. Patience was key.

July 2014

I successfully conducted two of my triathlon training weeks in the French Alps. During the planning stages it was obvious I should simply focus on one business activity (triathlon) rather than trying to attain pre-accident working and performance levels of consecutive cycle and triathlon training weeks. The recovery implications needed to be factored in based on the previous year's Grand Alps tour from Geneva to Nice.

It was great to be back coaching groups of triathletes again. Consideration and creativity helped me find adaptations in coaching delivery and guiding, instead of leading from the front on the roads or trails. My body coped well with the endurance training on consecutive days, improved recovery and less pain than the previous year. In many aspects, these were some of the best training camps I had delivered in the seven years since starting the training weeks in the French Alps. I had missed the personal engagement and detailed observation opportunities by not being able to ride, run and swim with my athletes. Another milestone had been reached. I was excited about developing another stage by the following summer on the long 10- to 12-hour drive from the French Alps to London.

Recovery cycle, two to four weeks:

To assist adaptation from a training progression or increase in duration, such as consecutive day training load

>> Reduce training volume.

>> Reduce training intensity.

>> Train 'little and often' as you feel.

>> Be guided by levels of motivation to train, fatigue and pain from injury sites.

>> Non-impact sport training – swimming, walking, strength and conditioning, yoga and Pilates.

>> Specific physiotherapy for injury sites.

>> Regular sports massage.

>> Quality nutrition, ensure protein intake is adequate and choose non-refined carbohydrates.

» Review effective areas of rehab and implement key exercises or sessions.

» Make connections by measuring progress from previous stage and improve confidence.

August 2014

Some rest and recovery was required throughout August, reducing my training volume with shorter sessions and a focus on strength, function and swimming. My high motivation levels from another significant breakthrough led me to start looking at the race calendar. I was keen to toe a start line at a local 10K race, building on the 5K events in the spring.

Reducing my time on the bike and prioritising a focus on strength, swimming and running had restored my back pain levels to marginal. I decided to stay off the bike in the short term and note the effect on pain levels in my lower back and pelvis. The assumption that the running impact was causing the ongoing low-level pain from my injuries was challenged, and there was one way to find out. My road bike was retired to the garage at the end of the summer although I continued to use my vintage commuter bike for short, local trips.

I gradually started to incorporate short tempo intervals into my run training and enjoyed the lift in pace. My run form and technique felt consolidated as I approached threshold running speed, and it seemed a familiar place, although my conditioning was limited to sustain it.

With the development of more speed I became more aware of my right leg seeming longer than the left. This was a regular observation in yoga and strengthening sessions in the gym. When sitting on the floor with legs extended my right knee was clearly offset 3 to 4 centimetres below the left knee. When standing my posture asymmetry was obvious in the level of my hip bones and slight curvature to the right through my spine and neck. In movement, particularly running, this caused frequent tripping on flat terrain.

My left leg always sounded and seemed to land more heavily than the right. I had ongoing pain in the left knee during and after easy paced runs as a result of the pelvis being aligned differently.

I had been cautious not to progress duration or speed while there was pain from any part of my body. The issue of pelvis misalignment and leg-length discrepancy culminated in a nasty fall one Sunday morning on an endurance run. Luckily I was on a soft equestrian trail and at low speed. I tripped over my right foot and landed heavily on both knees, hands and elbows, practically on all fours. The grazed wound on my right knee was significantly larger and deeper than the left, evidencing the hip alignment problem. My palms, elbows and wrists were all grazed, too. It was a long, painful limp home that day! I needed many weeks to let the knees repair and heal, subsequently returning to light running with two painful knees which restricted any ambitious thoughts around progression.

Sunday 20 September 2014

Many weeks later I lined up on Wimbledon Common to run a local 10K, ready to begin my first race in three years. The starter briefed us with the course layout, laps and marshals. Then we were off!

I found myself running behind the lead pack of 10 men and settled into what felt like a sustainable pace and rhythm. After the first lap at 5 kilometres I looked at my watch showing a 20:45 split on the display. This was a surprise. I hoped I could continue running at what felt like a sustainable but challenging pace.

Approaching the 6-kilometre mark and something happened in my lower back. I started to feel a little strange around the sacrum area. My left hamstring started to tighten and have an impact on my stride rhythm and length. The words of the hospital consultant, 'you will not be able to run again', echoed in my head. I switched focus back to my body and asked the question. Could I keep going for another 4 kilometres?

By relaxing the pace a little I managed to run the final 3 to 4 kilometres at a little easier pace, finishing just outside the top 10 overall in 42:03. I was delighted. I hadn't been overtaken in the final 5 kilometres and had held my position within the group at the front; my pace had slowed a little but not a huge amount. Afterwards I found it amazing how my body tuned back into a natural rhythm, as I began running with the mindset of a 'race head' on. I was awarded quite possibly the largest trophy I have ever received for winning an event in the past 12 years. Although overwhelmed by the size and scale of it earned in a little over 40 minutes, I smiled at the scale of recovery the silverware symbolised.

I spent the next few weeks in another recovery cycle, attending physiotherapy to work through the sacrum, lower back, and hamstring issue. Having regular sports massages, stretching and strengthening helped to coax the tightness and pain referring into my hamstring and lower back to relatively pain free. Low-intensity training provided the familiar routine and confidence that experiencing pain, soreness and fatigue was not a setback, instead part of the adaptation process. The regular challenge of finding new levels in function and performance alongside injury management as a continued adaptation cycle was now a new dimension in my life.

I looked forward to planning a return to multisport and triathlon in 2015.

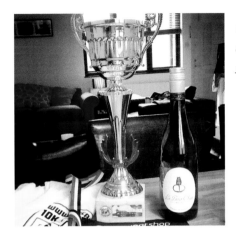

Ignore your performance decline post injury and focus instead at training from where you are, towards your aims or targets.

Paul Newsome's advice for resuming training to return to competitive form:

Personally I set myself a very long-term plan of returning to full health. Once I had gone through the major rehabilitation work that needed to be done (and continues to be part of my training plan to this day), I decided to start back at what seemed like a ridiculously low level. The only goal was for each session to be better than the last, and it was.

My goals and target times were very achievable, but even knowing that this was an 'easy route' – and one which was much easier than I would have otherwise chosen had it not been for the surgery – it filled me with positivity and motivation knowing that I was getting better step by step, day by day.

I wrote the goals down and sent them to a training partner of equal ability who guffawed a bit at how easy they were, but I've stuck to them, and though they had a much looser focus, I'm now swimming 2 minutes per kilometre quicker than them as a result. Consistency for the long term is what counts, and this is precisely what I did and exactly how I'd encourage others to approach a post-surgery rehabilitation period.

Paul Newsome, *owner of SwimSmooth, 2013 Manhattan Island Marathon Swim champion*

The start line – toeing it again:

Belief

Drawing on experience of competitive sport and training, the body can and will adapt with the right conditions. All you need is time, patience and consistency. Investing in a rehabilitation plan will perhaps result in a more balanced, better-functioning body than pre-injury. It is an opportunity to recreate a better version of yourself that you may not have otherwise had. The experience invested in your sport pre-injury will not evaporate in a matter of days, weeks, months, even years on the recovery trail.

Consistency

Be consistent with all aspects of training, nutrition and recovery or rest. Challenge the body without overreaching; monitor by checking in with daily stretching and movement rituals. Go beyond set physiotherapy exercises, and complete them every day. Be creative to seek progression where and when you need it. Apply attention to detail in planning to ensure you remain motivated and challenged.

Expectations

Keep expectations realistic. Transition back from participation level to competitive level in order to manage expectations and gradually increase the level of challenge. Measure improvement based on short, medium and long-term progress from the level you were previously.

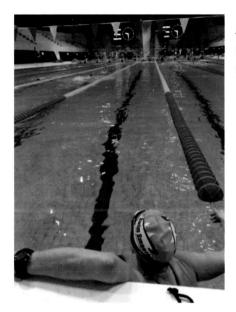

Appreciate the journey back to multisport training and competition: it can take many routes.

'The perspective from the top of the mountain does not take into account the challenges required on the ascent. Don't set your goals with a top-down mentality.

As you climb to reach the summit, remember to appreciate the views back towards where you started. Work upwards from your start point as there are many ways to reach the top!'

CHAPTER 10:
PRE-TRAINING PLANS AND SESSIONS

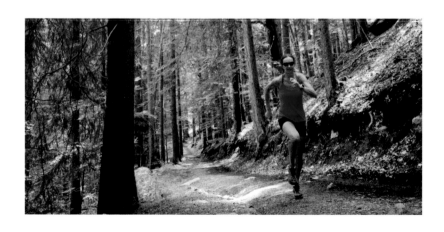

Pre-training

Pre-training aims to provide a foundation to build from after injury or a long training break through exercise rehabilitation. For a multisport athlete this involves a balance of strengthening, physiotherapy and light aerobic intensity training in each discipline. An athlete recovering from multiple injuries may benefit from a staged approach, focusing on one discipline at a time to comprehensively recover movement patterns and strength in one sport before incorporating another one or two sports.

The phase between physiotherapy to recover range of movement from the acute effects of injury and full training can be lengthy in duration lack the same structure as a training plan and be full of setbacks. A conservative approach and gradual increase in training load should be balanced with ongoing strengthening, stabilising and management.

Always ensure that you have completed your physiotherapy plan and sought medical advice specific to recovering from your individual injuries. Once you have been given the all-clear to begin low-intensity exercise and movement, introducing pre-training in stages will effectively facilitate adaptation back to multisport.

Aims of pre-training:

>> Provide a foundation of aerobic conditioning for the athlete to resume training

>> Improve balance, co-ordination, muscular strength and endurance

>> Increase joint mobility and range of movement

>> Establish optimal muscle performance and movement patterning specific to the athlete's sport or sports

>> Re-establish or improve and develop neuromuscular control

>> Improve postural stability and address asymmetrical issues or compensation post injury

>> Restore the athlete's confidence by connecting their sport and training at a manageable level for their stage of progress and recovery

Table 4

MULTISPORT STAGED RECOVERY TIMELINE PRE-TRAINING				
Stage 1 1-3 months post injury	Physiotherapy	Hydrotherapy	Walking	Swimming	Activation exercises, stretching
Stage 2 2-12 months post injury	Physiotherapy	Pool rehabilitation Pool walking Pool running	Cycling, aerobic and strength focused	Swimming	Strength and conditioning movement and activation exercises
	Yoga or Pilates	Walking	Running and cycling drills (low intensity)	Low-intensity running	Sports massage Fascia release as required around injury sites

Begin with stage 1 sessions, starting from suggested lower range of duration on the main set after the warm-up. Increase the duration gradually over two to five sessions per week, depending on implementation of a single- or multisport approach.

Progression to stage 2 will depend on the reaction from injury sites and reduction in pain levels. Remain in stage 1 until improvement is noted and injuries have been assessed for recovery.

Work on range of movement and activation of muscle groups during the sessions. It is not important to be working at high intensity or aiming to complete more distance each session. Instead, work with the training metrics of time, rhythm and rate of perceived effort.

Advance to stage 2 when injury pain and movement patterns have improved on the recommendations of physiotherapist or medical advice to resume light exercise.

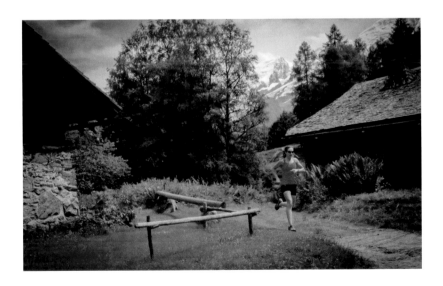

Pool walking to pool running

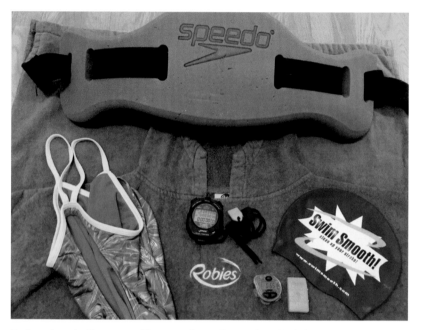

Equipment required for water walking or running sessions: Pool running belt, stopwatch or pool clock, timing devices that emit a regular beep: Wetronome or Tempo Trainer, optional heart rate monitor

Training metrics:

» Heart rate (HR)

» Cadence as SPM (strides per minute); count left or right leg revolutions per minute

» Time (minutes)

HR

Optional. If you have a HR monitor to provide feedback and are used to training with this feedback, use it. Apply your run training zones, if you have them from your pre-injury training. Aim to work predominantly within zones 1 and 2 at aerobic endurance intensity at or below your lactate threshold <85% of your MHR (for running).

MHR – maximum heart rate: 220 – your age is not accurate enough for athletes due to the wide range of individual variation in trained or untrained runners, cyclists and swimmers. There will also be variation between cycling, running and swimming maximal HR. A true MHR can only be identified by performance testing or repeatable field tests and training sets.

If you haven't any specific run HR training zones, keep it simple and work with SPM instead.

SPM

To develop understanding of leg rhythm in strides per minute terms just takes a little time and practice. You can measure SPM intrinsically by counting and using the pace clock or extrinsically using a Wetronome or Tempo Trainer set to a given SPM rhythm.

Start by counting the number of times an identified leg (right or left) moves through a full revolution over 30 seconds and double it to work out your SPM.

Use the pool's swim pace clock, or if there isn't one available or easily sighted, set your watch to display time in minutes and seconds.

Form-focused tips:

» Wear a pool running belt.

» Try to run in the water as well as you would on land.

» Avoid leaning too far forward and utilise your core muscles to keep you upright in the water.

» Don't run for distance. It is very easy to try and focus on 'how many lengths am I doing?' rather than maintaining good form. You really shouldn't cover much more than 10 metres within a minute!

Warm-up

Once you are in the water with the belt on, start moving into deep water. Find a steady rhythm and don't try and race anyone swimming in the lanes beside you!

Begin the following form check from the feet up to your head and shoulders.

Spend a minute or two focusing on each aspect:

Feet – keep them as flat as you can; don't point your toes. You really don't want to be scooting up and down the pool using your feet as paddles or to lift you up as if you're treading water.

Legs – aim for a circular motion. Focus on the front of the lift, using your core to engage the leg forward from the body. There should be a 90-degree angle through hips and knees.

Drive through the full leg circle to extend behind you and recover. Keep the movement nice and even; you might discover a weakness in one leg related to your injury or movement compensation. Practise some high-knee lift drills and leg flicks behind you to exaggerate the movement and activate all the major muscle groups as dynamic stretches.

Core and lower back – keep this activated and strong; use breathing to help stay in rhythm with your running. Think about it being the central point everything will pivot from.

Upper back, chest – keep them above your core and centre of gravity above your legs. Imagine you are running on land, where would you feel comfortable leaning - back, forward or in the middle? Try doing this to work out where you need to be to be balanced.

Shoulders – keep these nice and loose to let your arms drive through; again don't let them take you too far forward. Feel your ribs gliding back and forth as you drive your arms forward and back. The resistance of the water makes this an excellent strengthening exercise for the shoulders and upper back, too!

Arms – keep both driving through the water strongly in time with your legs. When you get tired use the elbows to keep the rhythm going. Pulling the elbows back behind the body helps the opposite leg to extend forward. Your triceps and biceps will feel the workload, too; toned arms are one of the many benefits of pool running!

Keep your fingers and hand relaxed, not clenched or open and pulling through the water. Lead the arm forward and back with the hand and elbow; avoid crossing in front of the body.

Neck and head – the head is relatively heavy, so keep looking forward and not down. Your neck shouldn't feel strained; if it is, bring your head back in alignment with your shoulders and back to achieve neutral spine. Turn your head to look in the direction you are going as you turn, when changing direction. If you are practising pool walking or running in a standard pool lane, you will need to alternate directions where possible.

HR – if using

Check your HR monitor and see what your HR is doing. You should observe a gradual increase into aerobic endurance training zones (zones 1 and 2) if you have spent a minute or two on each of the exercises.

SPM

Complete your warm-up by completing 5-10 x 30-second efforts, increasing your cadence to 70 spm. Aim to count 35 revolutions per leg over 30 seconds. The pool pace clock is useful for monitoring SPM. Position yourself within a lane to complete the main set of your session where you can easily sight the clock at regular intervals.

Table 5

Stage 1	**Pool walking 1**
Weeks 1-4	Warm-up: 10 minutes form focused
	Main set: 2-5 x 2 minutes at 60-69 rpm + 1 minute easy recovery <60 rpm
	Start at the lower end of the range (2 repeats of 2 minutes) and gradually progress towards the upper range guide (5 repeats of 2 minutes) as injury pain and movement range dictate. Spend at least one week at each increase, repeating the same session.
	Cool-down: Easy 5 minutes. Perform exaggerated slow circles with each leg to dynamically stretch out muscle groups; point and flex toes and feet. Float on back and scull arms back and forth to stretch out shoulders.
	Duration: 20-30 minutes

Stage 1 Weeks 5-8	**Pool walking 2** Warm-up: 10 minutes form focused Main set: 2-5 x 5 minutes at 60-69 rpm + 1 minute easy recovery <60 rpm Start at the lower end of the range (3x5 min) and gradually progress towards the upper range guide (5x5 min) as injury pain and movement range dictate. Spend at least one week at each increase, repeating the same session. Cool-down: Easy 5 minutes. Perform exaggerated slow circles with each leg to dynamically stretch out muscle groups; point and flex toes and feet. Float on back and scull arms backwards and forwards to stretch out shoulders. Duration: 40-45 minutes
Stage 2 Weeks 9-12	**Pool running 1** Warm-up: 10 minutes, establish 60 spm and work through form check from feet, legs, hips, core, lower back, upright posture, hands, arms, shoulders, neck and head. Main set: 6-10 x 3 minutes at 70-79 rpm + 1 minute jog recoveries at 60 rpm Cool-down: Easy 5 minutes, dynamically stretch out muscle groups with exaggerated slow leg circles. Finish with a few minutes kicking on your back with the belt. Duration: 44-55 minutes

Stage 2 Weeks 12-15	**Pool running 2** Warm-up: 10 minutes, establish 60 spm and work through form check from feet, legs, hips, core, lower back, upright posture, hands, arms, shoulders, neck and head. Main set: 4-7 x 5 minutes at 70-79 rpm + 1 minute jog recovery at 60 rpm Cool-down: Easy 5 minutes, dynamically stretch out muscle groups with exaggerated slow leg circles. Finish with a few minutes kicking on your back with the belt. Duration: 40-57 minutes
Stage 2 Weeks 15-20	**Pool running 3** Warm-up: 10 minutes form focus, establish rhythm at 60-69 spm Main set: 7-10 x 3 minutes at 80-85 rpm, +1 minute jog recovery at 60 rpm Cool-down: Easy 5-10 minutes, dynamically stretch out muscle groups with slow and exaggerated forward and reverse circles. Finish with a few minutes kicking on your front and back using the belt as a float for support (remove from waist). Duration: 42-60 minutes
Stage 2 Weeks 21-24	**Pool running 4** Warm-up: 10 minutes form focus, establish rhythm at 60-69 spm 4-6 x 6 minutes at 85-89 rpm, +1 minute jog recovery at 60 rpm Cool-down: Easy 5-10 minutes, dynamically stretch out muscle groups with slow and exaggerated forward and reverse circles. Finish with a few minutes kicking on your front and back using the belt as a float for support (remove from waist). Duration: 48-60 minutes

Water walking and running SPM values for triathletes:

Table 6

SPM (STRIDES PER MINUTE)	PACE (LAND EQUIVALENT)	RPE (RATE OF PERCEIVED EXERTION [1-10])
50-59	Brisk walk at 6.5 kph	1-2 Very light
60-69	Easy jog, recovery pace between intervals Aerobic threshold pace	3-4 Light
70-79	Tempo pace Half marathon pace	5-6 Somewhat hard
80-89	10 km to 5 km race pace Threshold pace	7-8
90-95 Not suitable for pre-training stages	Intervals at 400 m-1600 m pace Anaerobic effort	9-10

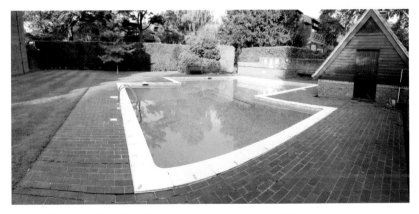

Implementing successful water walking or running sessions in a small pool

Cycle pre-training

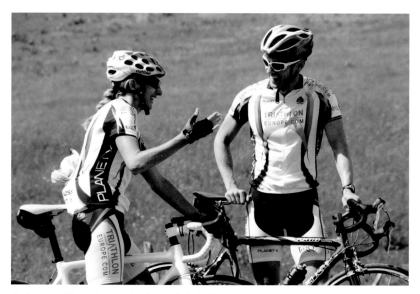

Cycle pre-training aims to develop technical skills, handling and confidence from an indoor environment back to the road outside.

Begin by identifying an optimal cycle setup to support the athlete's stage of recovery and particular injuries. Indoor cycling options offer greater flexibility in adjusting rider position such as gym bike, spin bike or a stationary trainer with suitable road bike. Assess all options available to identify the least painful or aggravating to injury sites.

Stage 1 can start once the athlete has had medical advice to proceed; depending on injury this may be one to three months into the recovery process. Cycle pre-training can be integrated as part of a staged rehabilitation plan, after a swim pre-training phase has been completed and before a running pre-training phase is begun. A return to multisport could be staged over 6 to 12 months, depending on how serious the injuries were and the rate of recovery.

Repeat the same session duration each week. Make gradual increases week on week, increasing duration and effort as injury pain decreases. Support the body's cycling adaptation with physiotherapy, strength and conditioning and deep tissue massage to manage reactions in and around injury sites.

Aim to progress in stage 2 with the introduction of outdoor cycling. This may be influenced by seasonal conditions and can be continued indoors if desired. It is not essential, although some implications for regaining cycling technical skills, confidence and handling will need to be planned in at a later stage. A specific cycling training week can assist to fast track these skills in a different environment to that which the athlete would usually train.

Training metrics:
>> Heart rate (HR) optional

>> Cadence as RPM (revolutions per minute) count left or right leg revolutions per minute

>> Power (watts) optional

>> Time (minutes)

RPM
Most indoor cycles will have cadence displayed on the monitor if in a gym environment. On an indoor cycle without a bike computer measuring the crank revolutions per minutes, count your left or right leg pedalling over 60 seconds to calculate your pedalling cadence. Over time this will become more intuitive, and the athlete will be able to identify their optimal cadence range where they are most efficient. Use HR and power to identify efficiency range on a cadence ramp test.

Warm-up

Pedal at low intensity and comfortable effort for 10 to 15 minutes. Start on an easy resistance for 5 minutes and gradually increase gears and resistance every 2 minutes, maintaining your perceived optimal cadence.

As you work through the warm-up process, assess the following:

Feet – note whether you are pedalling toes down, heels up or with flat feet horizontal to the floor. Aim to distribute the muscular effort evenly through both legs; use a pedal scan on Wattbike to assess and correct if a lower-body injury is causing an obvious imbalance left and right.

Legs – aim for a circular motion with effort engaging solely from the hips and torso. Reduce any bouncing on the saddle when pedalling a light resistance by engaging less of the quads to push down and more of the glutes to drive the leg around the pedal stroke.

Core and lower back – Resting lightly on the handlebars, use your core to keep the spine neutral. Engage the core on lower gear work and avoid moving from side to side on the saddle as you progress through the warm-up to lower cadence values which simulate climbing.

Shoulders – keep shoulder blades lightly squeezed back and down to avoid rounding through the upper back. Utilise a change in position to stretch out shoulders and back on recoveries. Experiment with more aerodynamic positions on the drops or tribars (if fitted) and more upright on the hoods or handlebars to simulate hill climbing.

Arms – elbows relaxed and not overextended with hands resting lightly on the handlebars. Avoid being too stretched out on your bike setup.

Neck and head – look up and forward, occasionally looking from side to side to check range of movement relating to any upper-body injury or shoulder issue.

HR – if using

You should observe a gradual increase into aerobic endurance training zones (zones 1 and 2) if you have spent a minute or two on each of the exercises.

RPM

Complete your warm-up by completing 3-5 x 20-second efforts increasing your cadence to 90 to 100 rpm. Spin recovery at 60 to 70 rpm for up to 2 minutes in between. Maintain controlled pedalling and symmetry in technique and form.

Table 7

Stage 1 Weeks 1-4	**Cycling intro 1** Warm-up: 10-15 minutes, light gear or resistance If in pain from injuries, remain at warm-up duration until this becomes manageable before starting stage 1. Main set: 1 minute at 100-105 rpm 1 minute at 90-95 rpm 1 minute at 80-85 rpm 1 minute at 70-75 rpm 1 minute at 60-65 rpm Progression each week: From 1-minute intervals to 90 seconds, 2 minutes, 3 minutes on each cadence range. If using HR, note which cadence values are most efficient – HR remains in aerobic zone 1 or 2 range (<85% MHR). Observe where spikes occur and perceived effort is high. Cool-down: Easy 5 minutes, at perceived optimal cadence Duration: 20-35 minutes

Stage 1 Weeks 5-8	**Cycling intro 2** Warm-up: 10-15 minutes, light gear or resistance Main set: 1 minute at 100-105 rpm 1 minute at 90-95 rpm 1 minute at 80-85 rpm 1 minute at 70-75 rpm 1 minute at 60-65 rpm 1 minute at 70-75 rpm 1 minute at 80-85 rpm 1 minute at 90-95 rpm 1 minute at 100-105 rpm Progression each week: From 1-minute intervals to 90 seconds, 2 minutes, 3 minutes on each cadence range. If using HR, note which cadence values are most efficient – HR remains in aerobic zone 1-2 range (<85% MHR). Observe where spikes occur and perceived effort is high. Cool-down: Easy 5 minutes, at perceived optimal cadence Duration: 30-45 minutes
Stage 2 Weeks 9-12	**Cycle session 1** Warm-up: 10-15 minutes, light gear or resistance working systematically through a form check, noting improvements or ongoing tightness or injury restrictions Main set: 5 minutes at optimal cadence (OC) 2-minute spin recovery 2.5 minutes at 70-75 rpm 2-minute spin recovery 5 minutes at optimal cadence 2-minute spin recovery 2.5 minutes at 100-105 rpm Progression each week: + 5 minutes at OC + 2.5 minutes at 60-65 rpm alternating seated and standing climbing positions every 30 seconds + 5 minutes at OC Cool-down: 5-10 minutes easy spin Duration: 45-60 minutes

Stage 2 Weeks 12-15	**Cycle session 2** Warm-up: 10-15 minutes, light gear or resistance working systematically through a form check, noting improvements or ongoing tightness or injury restrictions Main set: 4-6 x 6 minutes at aerobic intensity (zone 2 HR ~80-85% MHR or L2w) + 1-minute spin recoveries Work at different cadence ranges on each 6-minute interval, from 60 rpm through to 100 rpm. At 60-65 rpm, alternate seated and standing every 60 seconds. Optional progression could include a longer endurance ride once per week to 65-75 minutes (zones 1 to 2 HR) in addition to the increase in main set repeats on subsequent weekly sessions. Aim to ride endurance rides at an aerobic, conversational pace, working on technical skills, climbing, descending, handling and confidence on the road. Cool-down: 5-10 minutes easy spin Duration: 50-60 minutes
Stage 2 Weeks 15-20	**Cycle session 3** Warm-up: 10-15 minutes, include 6-8 minutes of single-leg drill work on a light resistance. Note left and right dominance. Main set: 3-4 x 7.5 minutes split intervals as aerobic endurance into tempo effort. Work for 5 minutes at zone 2 HR/ L2w and increase effort into zone 3 HR (~90% MHR)/ L3w for remaining 2.5 minutes of each interval. + 2.5-minute spin recoveries at 100-110 rpm, focusing on pedalling efficiency. Optional progression could also include a longer endurance ride once per week to 65-75 minutes (zones 1-2 HR) in addition to the increase in main set repeats on subsequent weekly sessions. Aim to ride endurance rides at an aerobic, conversational pace, working on technical skills, climbing, descending, handling and confidence on the road. Cool-down: 5-10 minutes easy spin Duration: 55-60 minutes

Stage 2 Weeks 21-24	**Cycling session 4** Warm-up: 10-15 minutes, include 6-8 minutes of single-leg drill work on a light resistance. Note left and right dominance. Main set: 8-10 x 3 minutes at tempo effort zone 3 HR (~90% MHR)/ L3w + 1-minute spin recoveries at 100-110 rpm, focusing on pedalling efficiency. Optional progression could include a longer endurance ride once per week to 65-75 minutes (zones 1-2 HR) in addition to the increase in main set repeats on subsequent weekly sessions. Aim to ride endurance rides at an aerobic, conversational pace, working on technical skills, climbing, descending, handling and confidence on the road. Cool-down: 5-10 minutes easy spin Duration: 55-60 minutes

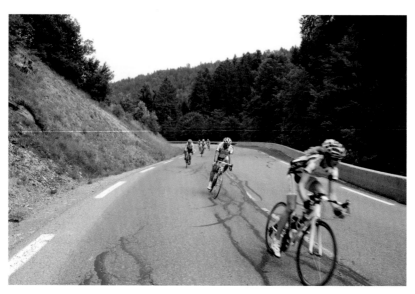

A training week away from the athlete's training environment is an effective way to develop confidence and technical skills.

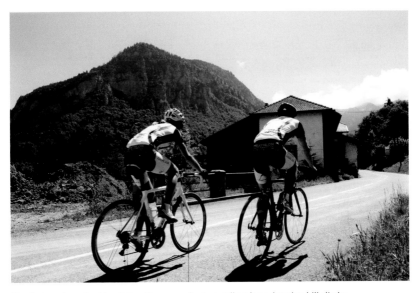

Developing strength at low intensities on moderate gradient long-duration hill climbs

Swim pre-training

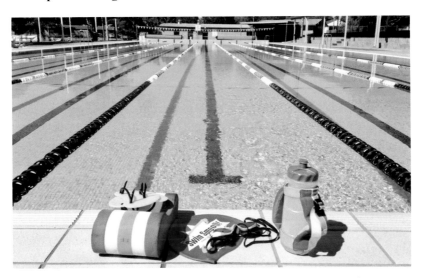

Use training aids such as fins, pull buoy and sculling paddles for swim pre-training sessions.

Swimming pre-training is excellent rehabilitation for lower-body injuries and can be implemented early in a staged rehabilitation process for triathletes, prior to reintroducing cycling and running.

For athletes with shoulder or neck and upper-back injuries, note the progressions using leg kick efficiency drills. Athletes with leg and hip injuries can work more on the upper-body drills and techniques initially.

Ensure that the physiotherapy process or medical advice has confirmed sufficient recovery post injury or surgery to rotate the arms before starting stage 1.

Each session incorporates a specific technical element:

» Body and leg position

» Body rotation and alignment

» Propulsion – the catch and pull phases

» Breathing and head position

Stage 1 provides time guides to work through the session. Progression to stage 2 relies on injuries responding well to swim pre-training, developing 'feel for the water' and pain reduction. Repeat stage 1 if required.

Table 8

Stage 1	**Swimming intro session 1 – Body and leg position**
Weeks 1-4	2-3 minutes kicking on front, back or sides with leading arm extended underwater (fins optional). Aim to elongate legs and kick from hips with toes pointed + 60-second rest.
	2-3 minutes sculling. Use pull buoy between thighs or knees to maintain body and leg position horizontally to the water surface + 60-second rest.
	2-3 minutes doggy paddle (fins optional). Practice with head in the water to ensure neck, spine and hips are neutrally aligned + 60-second rest.
	2-3 minutes kicking on front, back or sides (fins optional). Aim to elongate legs and kick from hips with toes pointed + 60-second rest.
	Progression over 4 weeks – repeat chosen or all session elements through once more.
	Duration: 8-24 minutes
Stage 1	**Swimming intro session 2 – Propulsion**
Weeks 5-8	5-6 minutes kicking on front, back or sides with leading arm extended underwater (fins optional). Work on continuous exhalation with head immersed on front and sides, looking down at pool floor (neutral spine). Optional – alternate with lengths of freestyle during each drill sequence. + 60-second rest
	5-6 minutes sculling (with pull buoy). Develop proprioception of forearm use and maintain flexion in wrist as you move the water side to side. Keep head immersed and lift to breathe in, exhaling continuously. Optional – alternate with lengths of freestyle during each drill sequence. + 60-second rest
	5-6 minutes doggy paddle with fins or pull buoy. Aim to perform the freestyle stroke underwater without arm recovery or rotation of the shoulders. Keep head immersed and lift to breathe in, exhaling continuously. Optional – alternate with lengths of freestyle during each drill sequence. + 60-second rest
	Progression over 4 weeks – repeat the session elements through once more.
	Duration: 15-36 minutes

Stage 2	**Swim session 1 – Body rotation and alignment**
Weeks 9-12	Warm-up: 4-8 x 25 m as doggy paddle into freestyle (FS). Use a pull buoy or fins, optional. Work on rotation to both sides and FS, tap thigh as hand exits the water + 15 seconds.
	Main set: 4-8 x 50 m as kicking on front, back or sides with leading arm extended in front of shoulder. Retract shoulder blades to open chest throughout the kicking drill into FS +15 seconds.
	4-8 x 100 m as FS, work on hand entry in front of shoulders and finishing off the stroke with the diagonally opposite arm (tap thigh) + 30 seconds.
	Cool-down: 4 x 25 m easy, breaststroke or choice
	Progression: work through the increase in each set from 4 to 8 repeats of each distance.
	Total: 800 m to 1500 m
Stage 2	**Swim session 2 – Breathing and head position**
Weeks 12-15	Warm-up: 4-8 x 50 m FS +15-20 seconds
	Main set: 100-200 m PULL (with pull buoy); identify optimal head position during each length +30 seconds.
	200-300 m with fins. Kick on side with leading arm extended, breathing left side for one length, right side for one length + 30-60 seconds.
	100-200 m PULL maintaining bilateral breathing. Alternate breathing every 3 and 5 strokes each length. Work on consistent exhalation throughout + 30 seconds.
	200-300 m FS, consolidating breathing technique.
	Cool-down: 4 x 50 m choice strokes
	Progression: work through the increase in distance within each set, consolidating breathing technique.
	Total: 1000 m to 1600 m

Stage 2	**Swim session 3 – Body and leg position**
Weeks 15-20	Warm-up: 4 x 100 m FS +15-30 seconds Main set: 3-4 x 200 m as 25-50 m sculling drill or doggy paddle into 150-175 m FS. Working on optimising catch and pull to ensure water is pressed back with elbow high, ensuring body, hips and legs remain parallel to surface + 30-60 seconds. 3-5 x 100 m FS with fins, kicking on side or back 50 m into FS. Aim to kick from hips with legs straight and toes pointed + 15-30 seconds. Cool-down: 2-3 x 100 m choice strokes Progression: work through the increase in each set from 2 to 4 repeats of each distance. Total: 1200 m to 2000 m
Stage 2	**Swim session 4 – Propulsion**
Weeks 21-24	Warm-up: 4 x 100 m FS + 15-30 seconds Main set: 2 x 100 m (with fins) with single arm drill into FS. Work on correct positioning of fingertips below wrist and maintain elbow above wrist performing the pull phase to finish stroke to tap thigh +15-30 seconds. 8 x 50 m as 25-m sculling drill or 25-m doggy paddle into FS (use pull buoy). Use small, sculling paddles as desired for this set +30-60 seconds. 200 m FS, consolidating propulsion with optimal catch and pull, introduce slight increase in stroke rate rhythm in second 100 m (negative split) + 60 seconds. Cool-down: 2 x 100 m choice strokes Progression: repeat some or all elements of main set over the 4 weeks. Total: 1400 m to 2200 m

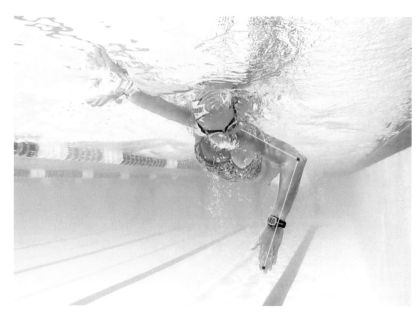

One of the benefits of swimming pre-training is a complete overhaul of swim technique and re-establishing a swimmer's 'feel for the water' before commencing full training.

Run pre-training

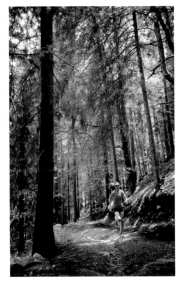

Off-road running is important for increased functional strength and stabilisation during pre-training.

Begin the return to jog plan at stage 1 of pre-training. The prerequisite for this phase is to build up to walking for 20 minutes at a comfortable speed. Progress your speed towards 6.5 kph. Once you can do this without aggravation or pain then you can progress to stage 1.

Progression to stage 2 relies on usual physiotherapy and medical advice, assessment of injury healing and pain from injury sites. Stage 1 may take further consolidation if the athlete sustained multiple injuries.

Incorporate off road, trails and sand surfaces for sessions during stage 2. Perform drills on grass or level, soft surfaces.

Training metrics:

>> Heart rate (HR) optional

>> Cadence as SPM (strides per minute) count left or right leg revolutions per minute

>> Time (minutes)

Table 9

Stage 1	**Return to jog programme levels 1-4**
Weeks 1-4	Level 1: Day 1: Walk 4 minutes, Jog 1 minute, Walk 4 minutes and so on until 20 minutes is completed. Day 2: Rest/Weights/Swim/Cycle Day 3: Walk 4 minutes/Jog 1 minute for 20 minutes Day 4: Rest/Weights/Swim/Cycle Progress when level 1 causes no aggravation or pain during or after session. Level 2: Day 5: Walk 3 minutes/Jog 2 minutes or 3.5/1.5 minutes for 20 minutes Day 6: Rest/Weights/Swim/Cycle Day 7: Walk 3 minutes/Jog 2 minutes or 3.5/1.5 minutes for 20 minutes Day 8: Rest/Weights/Swim/Cycle Progress when level 2 causes no aggravation or pain during or after session. Level 3: Day 9: Walk 2 minutes/Jog 3 minutes for 20 minutes Day 10:Rest/Weights/Swim/Cycle Day 11: Walk 2 minutes/Jog 3 minutes for 20 minutes Day 12: Rest/Weights/Swim/Cycle Progress when level 3 causes no aggravation or pain during or after session. Level 4: Day 13: Walk 1 minute/Jog 4 minutes for 20 minutes Day 14: Rest/Weights/Swim/Cycle Day 15: Walk 1 minute/Jog 4 minutes for 20 minutes Day 16: Rest/Weights/Swim/Cycle Progress when level 4 causes no aggravation or pain during or after session.

Stage 1 Weeks 5-8	**Return to jog programme levels 5-8**
	Level 5: Day 17: Jog 20 minutes Day 18: Rest/Weights/Swim/Cycle Day 19: Jog 20 minutes Day 20: Rest/Weights/Swim/Cycle
	Level 6: Increase 20-minute continuous jog to 3 days per week. Alternate with rest, weights, swimming or cycling in between running days.
	Level 7: Increase to 25 minutes on one run per week. Maintain the two other runs at 20 minutes. Alternate with rest, weights, swimming or cycling in between running days.
	Level 8: Increase to 25 minutes on 2-3 runs per week, as recovery or pain from injury sites dictates. Alternate with rest, weights, swimming or cycling in between running days.
Stage 2 Weeks 9-12	**Running session 1**
	Warm-up: 5 minutes brisk walking 5 minutes easy jog
	Main set: Run/walk for 20 minutes as 7-9 minutes jog, 1-3 minutes walk. Increase each week by 3-5 minutes, aiming to complete 2-3 run sessions per week. On alternate days rest, swim, bike or strength training.
	Cool-down: 2-5 minutes brisk walk or easy jog
	Duration: 30-45 minutes

Stage 2 Weeks 12-15	**Running session 2** Warm-up: 2-3 minutes brisk walking 3-5 minutes easy jog 3-5 minutes run drills and activation exercises Main set: 30-minute continuous jog in zones 1-2 HR (aerobic endurance). Increase main set each week by 2-3 minutes, incorporating walking breaks of up to 5 minutes if required by pain. If pain free, aim to complete 2-3 run sessions per week. On alternate days rest, swim, bike or strength training. Cool-down: 5-10 minutes brisk walk or easy jog Duration: 40-50 minutes
Stage 2 Weeks 15-20	**Running session 3** Warm-up: 2-3 minutes brisk walking 3-5 minutes easy jog 3-5 minutes run drills and activation exercises Main set: 35-40-minute continuous jog, in zones 1-2 HR (aerobic endurance). Progression: Complete one run per week as alternating jog for 15 minutes, walk for 5 minutes. On alternate days rest, swim, bike or strength training. Cool-down: 5-10 minutes brisk walk or easy jog Duration: 47-60 minutes

Stage 2	**Running session 4**
Weeks 21-24	Warm-up: 2-3 minutes brisk walking 3-5 minutes easy jog 3-5 minutes run drills and activation exercises
	Main set: 40-45-minute continuous jog in zones 1-2 HR (aerobic endurance). Progression: Complete one run per week as alternating jog for 15 minutes, walk for 5 minutes. On alternate days rest, swim, bike or strength training. Cool-down: 5-10 minutes brisk walk or easy jog
	Duration: 53-60 minutes

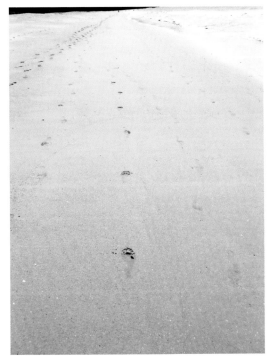

Sand running for gait analysis and improving form

EPILOGUE:
COMEBACK RACE

Top speed: 55 kph
Elevation gain: 190 m
Distance: 53.5 km

Windsor Triathlon, 14 June 2015

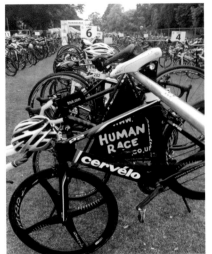

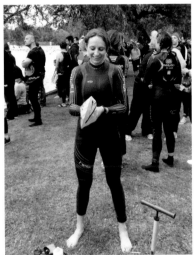

Bike racked pre-race at the Windsor Triathlon 2015

Before the swim start at my first race in nearly four years

I gazed at the downstream stretch of the River Thames, arms purposefully sculling the water in front of me at the start of the first Olympic distance wave of the Windsor Triathlon 2015. I felt calm and ready. I could feel the gentle river current tugging me past the start line. Equally keen to get underway I waited to be given the 10-second countdown to the race start. I started my 'lucky' race watch so I could go as soon as I heard the sound of the klaxon.

Familiar movement patterns and psychological preparations had returned in the days leading up to the race. It was like the four years away from the sport of triathlon had passed in the blink of an eye. Getting reunited with my old race kit and equipment had provoked memories of many a great performance and lots of fun times. It was great to be back on a start line again and I shivered with excitement.

Then the klaxon came. Simultaneous splashing erupted around me. We were off. I settled into a fast rhythm, using my legs to kick and maintain clear water at the front of the wave start. Within a minute or two I could see no other swimmers around me at all. I settled into a steadier rhythm and breathing pattern of every 3/2/3/2 strokes so I could navigate easily using the river bank and swim buoys in the middle of the river. I could feel the faster-moving water in the gentle current and intended to make good use of it by remaining in the middle of the river as far as possible.

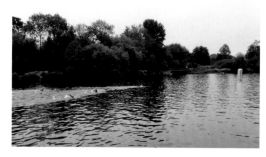

After 1000 m I reached the turn-around point and the kayakers directed me around the sweeping turn near the Eton bridge. I was the first triathlete onto the newly planned Olympic distance swim course. I gauged my lead as I headed back up the river to the exit approximately 500 m away – I was a good way ahead. Unfortunately a slight navigational error occurred at the swim exit. I missed the turn, ended up swimming further upstream, nearly colliding with some sprint distance competitors, before correcting myself. I lost my lead but made my exit and the run into T1 feeling strong with an excellent swim behind me.

Leading through the first 100 m of the Windsor Triathlon swim start

Swim: 23:47
Position 12 (overall), 2nd in age group

Reaching the transition area, I could not stop smiling when I saw my boyfriend Steve leaping up and down excitedly near my racked race bike. I could hear him long before I saw him, conveying bundles of positive energy. I was soon disappearing with my bike onto the long barefoot run out to the start of the bike course. I thought back to our lake swim the day before and recognised that, when his race started later that morning, he would probably love the new swim course as much as I did.

A smooth transition onto the bike, feet seamlessly finding their way into the bike shoes, and I got the bike up to speed. I could not take the smile off my face as I pedalled the bike up to race speed. The hum of my race wheels, the aerodynamic position perched on the front of the race saddle and the strength and energy being generated to turn the pedals felt amazing.

Within a few kilometres I heard a motorbike riding alongside and just behind me and realised I was being accompanied as the first competitor out onto the Olympic distance course.

I glanced at my Garmin and noted the bike speed around 35-38 kph. Accident impact speed... This thought connected but didn't daunt, instead it spurred me to keep the power on. I felt safe as I passed Sprint distance competitors at a significantly faster speed. The motorbike marshal sped ahead of me to clear the road of other competitors so I could pass by fast!

And then eventually I was on my own on the course after 20 km and left to tune into how sweetly the bike travelled. I uttered a number of silent 'thank-yous' to acknowledge how comfortably strong I felt. My back, sacrum, hips, shoulder and neck were all connected, painlessly doing a great job of generating power to the pedals. I couldn't believe it.

By the turn-around point of the bike course on Drift Road, I realised how far my lead had extended. It seemed I was about 2 kilometres ahead of the next competitor in my wave start. I rolled through the rest of the course, taking an energy gel before I whizzed down the only exhilarating descent beside the Windsor Great Park. The blurred sense of speed was exciting. I couldn't wait to get onto the run course.

Bike: 1:11:25
Position 4 (overall), 1st in age group

Arriving into T2 was always one of the technical parts of a race that I most enjoyed. Pedalling barefoot, feet on top of shoes, balancing on one pedal and timing the jump off with minimal bike speed reduction brought a fun element to any race, no matter how important it was. I swapped my bike and helmet for long compression socks and trainers and headed out onto the run course.

The three little climbs up to Windsor Castle awaited on the looped 10K course which had also been revamped for the 25th anniversary race. This was a part of the race I had always relished; however, I had suffered from a troublesome calf in the weeks leading up to the race and therefore opted for a conservative pace.

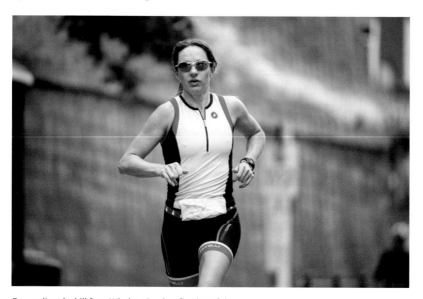

Descending the hill from Windsor Castle – first lap of the run course

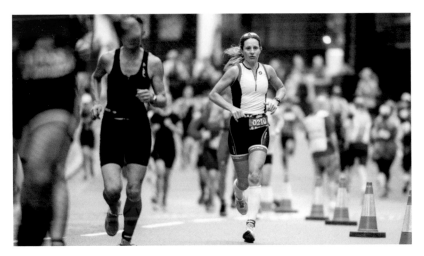

Final lap of the run course, in the lead

Every stride was uncomfortable and I experimented with forefoot and heel landing to reduce the pain levels as I ran the three laps. It wasn't ideal but gave me the opportunity to recognise many athletes I had worked with or coached over the years who were out on the course. We exchanged high fives, waves or thumbs up as we passed each other on the out and back sections of the run course.

Managing emotions became more of a challenge as I neared the finish. My former coach Spencer Smith was at the top of the hill on the last lap, and his words of encouragement left me making connections to some of the great races when he had coached me.

Seemingly on autopilot I made my way down the long finishing straight of the Windsor Triathlon. My mind was a long way from the race course and it was hard to hold back some tears of sheer delight as I crossed the finish line. Nothing worthwhile in life is ever easy and to progress through the stages of mobility, weight bearing, repairing the body, functional movement, multisport training, fatigue management and finally into competitive shape to get back on track has been the most rewarding experience of my life so far. A new chapter has successfully begun!

Run: 46:16
Position 22 (overall), 3rd in age group

Overall time:
2:29:28
Overall 7th, 1st in age group by a 12-minute clear winning margin

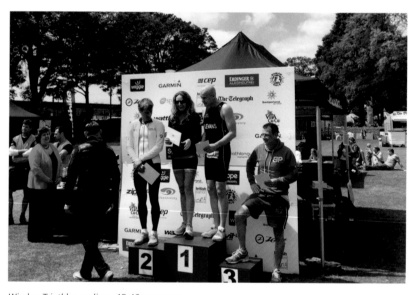

Windsor Triathlon podium, 45-49 age group

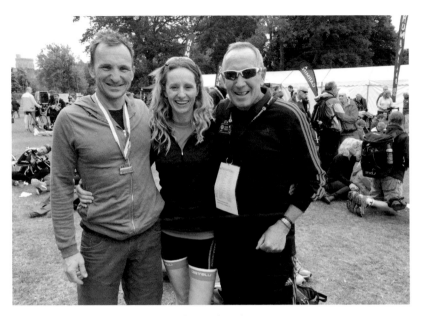

Celebrating post race with partner Steve Hobson and coach Steve Trew

CREDITS

Cover:	Andreas Reuel
Copyediting:	Elizabeth Evans
Layout and typesetting:	Andreas Reuel

PHOTO CREDITS

Cover:	©Simon Parker, SP Action Images
Inside:	©Triathlon Europe Ltd.: p. 177, 183, 186, 188, 189, 191, 192, 193, 197, 198, 200, 202, 203, 250, 256, 257, 262

**TRIΛTHLON
EUROPE**

©Rachel Morris: p. 15, 86

©Neil Brickley: p. 22

©Steve Folsom: p. 137, 216, 217

©Richard Melik, Freespeed: p. 163

©Paul Mercer: p. 238, 241, 263

©Dan Marshman: p. 237

©Simon Parker: p. 169, 205, 206, 209

©Training Peaks: p. 118-119

©Garmin Connect: p. 33

©Parkrun: p. 229

©Steve Hobson: p. 269 & 270 bottom

©Simon Parker, SP Action Images: p. 272 & 273

©all other pictures by Fiona Ford

Graphics: ©Thinkstock/iStock/Zephyr18